LIVING YOUNG
32 HABITS OF AGELESS PEOPLE

LIVING YOUNG
32 HABITS OF AGELESS PEOPLE

Andy Troy, C.S.C.S.

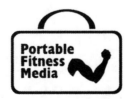

Disclaimer

This book is not intended as a substitute for the medical advice of a physician. The reader should regularly consult a physician in all matters related to his or her health, particularly in respect to any symptoms that may require diagnosis or medical attention.

Cover photo by Lina Jang

Illustrations by Brandon Li

ISBN-13: 978-0-9792081-0-2
ISBN-10: 0-9792081-0-6

Library of Congress Control Number: 2007921901

Portable Fitness Media LLC
1421 Sheepshead Bay Road #136
Brooklyn New York, 11235

Printed in the U.S.A.

*"The preservation of health is a duty. Few seem conscious
that there is such a thing as physical morality."*
—Herbert Spencer

Acknowledgments

I would like to thank the following people. Their knowledge and expertise have proven invaluable and they, like me, are part of what you are about to read.

Mary Lou Andre: Fashion Consultant

Joan Arnold: Certified Teacher of the Alexander Technique, Registered Yoga Teacher

Wendy Barreto: New York State Certified Massage Therapist

Kathy Browning: Feng Shui Practitioner

Richard Brennan: I.S.A.T.T., S.T.A.T., A.T.I., Certified Teacher of the Alexander Technique, Registered Yoga Teacher

Al Bumanis, MT-BC: AMTA Director of Communications (Music Therapy)

Michelle Cobey: the Delta Society (Pet Therapy)

Linda Feingold, MEd, MS, RD: Nutritionist

Mauro Hernandez: New York State Certified Massage Therapist

Joe Lupo: Fashion Consultant

Dr. Jane Pentz: Nutritionist

Dr. William Pezzello: Chiropractor

Viraj Santini: Bikram Yoga Instructor

Dr. Steven Simon: Dermatologist

Dr. Alcibiades Rodriguez: (Sleep Disorders)

Anne Taylor: Yoga Instructor

Missy Vinyard: Certified Teacher of the Alexander Technique

Jessica Wolf: Breathing Coordination Instructor

"Western medicine is like driving your car into a wall then taking it to the body shop to have it fixed. Eastern medicine is like getting your brakes fixed so that you don't drive into the wall."

—Andy Troy

Contents

Section III - After Work-Your Workout

Section IV - After Your Workout-Living it up then Winding Down

A Closing Word

Bibliography

Index

Weekly Chart

"All diseases run into one, old age."
—**Ralph Waldo Emerson**

Those Who Inspire

On September 14, 1889, in western Ecuador, Maria Esther Capovilla was born. That event in itself is in no way remarkable unless you consider that on August 14, 2006, she was still alive. More remarkable still is the fact that 116 year old Maria walked without assistance, had good vision, and was fully alert. She had outlived her husband by 56 years and enjoyed watching television, an invention whose birth she preceded by 36 years.

On a summer day in 1965, Leroy "Satchel" Paige took the mound for the final time, providing the Kansas City Athletics with three shutout innings. That feat in itself might not seem worth including in a list of great athletic accomplishments, unless you consider that on that date Paige, a Negro League legend, was believed to be 60 years of age.

On November 20, 1984, fitness guru Jack LaLanne celebrated his birthday in an unusual way. He did so by taking a mile-long swim while towing 70 rowboats filled with 70 people. Making the event even more unusual was the fact that on that date, Jack LaLanne was 70 years old.

On November 10, 2004, Roger Clemens was awarded his seventh Cy Young award, an honor bestowed each year on the pitcher in each league viewed as that season's most dominant. His statistics that year included a record of 18-4, 214 innings pitched, an earned run average of 2.98 and 218 strikeouts. What made this accomplishment all the more remarkable was that Roger Clemens was 42 years old.

In October 2005 *Walker, Texas Ranger: Trial by Fire* was released. It was a film featuring action star Chuck Norris who has been thrilling movie audiences with his martial arts expertise ever since moving from the ring to the silver screen. In the film Chuck kicks butt and defends the good guys from the bad guys in his customary style. As always he did all his own fight scenes, many of which would be challenging for men in their 30s. At the time the film was released, Chuck Norris was 65 years old.

On October 25, 2005, I was privileged to witness a reunion performance by Cream, one of the greatest rock and roll bands of all time. There were many memorable moments for me that night as I went about reliving my youth but perhaps the most remarkable was watching 66 year old Ginger Baker play the drums for over two hours without a break. His performance included a lengthy drum solo that would have put many 20 year olds to shame.

In the November 2005 edition of *Big* magazine, 61-year-old Lauren Hutton did something most 20-year-old women would not have the self confidence to do: a nude photo shoot. This was not an embarrassing miscalculation on her part. Instead, it was an example of a woman who knew she could compete favorably with those 40 years her junior.

"You end up as you deserve. In old age you must put up with the face, the friends, the health, and the children you have earned."
—Judith Viorst

Introduction

There is a disease more feared than all others. It affects men and women alike, causing every cell in the body to wither and die. It proves fatal in all cases and as yet there is no cure. That disease is called aging.

Youth is a fleeting thing, yet one we want very much to preserve. In spite of this our lives often lead us down a very different path. We eat the wrong foods, drink, smoke and work too much, exercise too little and get way too much sun. As badly as we want to preserve our youth, we seem to do everything in our power to cut it short. It's one of modern America's great paradoxes.

So much is made today of preventive medicine, something our ancestors clearly understood. Yet as much as we talk about the validity of the concept, we often do little to make it part of our lives.

Genetics are something we cannot control. In this book, I'm going to look at 32 things that we *can* control, factors that affect how well we age. Using today as your guide, read the following 32 questions and answer them honestly, then see how well you measure up. It might be an eye-opening experience that leads to seeing a younger, healthier you.

Some people may fare better when they can visualize how their day and week is progressing. For them, there is a weekly chart in the back of this book with each component listed. Feel free to make copies and post them somewhere visible, or if you prefer, take them with you. You can then check off each component, either as your day progresses or at the end of your day.

There is something you should keep in mind while reading this book. Though the chapters are set up individually, you will find many examples of synergy. That is because both wellness and the lack thereof have a domino effect. The world does not exist in a vacuum and what affects one aspect of the human condition is affected by many others. The healing properties of New Age music and aromatherapy combine to increase the effectiveness of massage. Both stretching and massage techniques can improve the flexibility necessary to attain and maintain proper posture. Exercise, especially yoga, and proper breathing techniques have an undeniable connection. This connection is something to always be aware of as you piece together the puzzle that is your health.

You will also find some chapters far longer than others. In these cases there was additional information that I felt would benefit you. The chapters on fitness are especially lengthy. Since the volume of both information and misinformation in regard to fitness is so vast, I felt that this was not only appropriate, but necessary.

You will notice that a full workout is part of this day. You won't necessarily go to the gym on a daily basis nor is it necessary for you to do so. On non-workout days simply skip that section and use the time that frees up to do something productive or just fun.

Finally, be aware that while much of the information listed is fact, I also make a number of recommendations. These are my opinions based on a combination of research and personal experience. Opinions vary and what helps one person may not help another, even if they have conditions that appear to be similar or even identical. Then again, if you didn't want my opinion you probably wouldn't be reading this book.

Below is a hypothetical day based on a 9-5 workday with a 45 minute commute. Keep in mind that it is just that: hypothetical. Everyone's life has different flexibilities as well as restrictions, many of which will force you to vary this schedule in one way or another. What this book gives you is a great deal of information on the things that can keep you young as well as a framework for how to put it all together. Read it, digest it, and let it work its way into your life.

All the best,

Andy

"You've got to work at living; dying is easy."
—Jack LaLanne

Section I:

BEFORE WORK

"Seek truth in meditation, not in moldy books. Look in the sky to find the moon, not in the pond."
—Persian proverb

"Meditation brings wisdom; lack of meditation leaves ignorance. Know well what leads you forward and what holds you back, and choose the path that leads to wisdom."
—Buddha

1   7 a.m.
Will You Meditate?

The alarm rings, the music comes on or your poodle licks your face, whatever it is that rouses you each morning makes its way into your consciousness. Your eyes open and you are ready to start your day. A good way to get it going in a positive direction is to meditate.

In the early seventies, when I was a teenager, the scent of the sixties was still in the air. People were experimenting with many ways of altering their consciousness, some healthy and some quite the opposite. It was then that my parents discovered a course called Mind Dimensions and Controls. Over the next four eight-hour days, the instructor, Roger Denim, exposed us to many New Age concepts, one of which was meditation. I found it highly beneficial, and though I lost contact with the school a few years later, I always remembered what I gained from the experience: a relaxed body and a less cluttered mind.

The years passed and my meditations became less frequent. I then found myself working in a highly stressful environment. There came a point where I knew I had to do something or there was going to be a problem. I decided to look to meditation to see what it could again offer me. I trekked down to the building where Mind Dimensions had been located only to find them gone without a trace. Disappointed, I decided to do some research, the results of which led me to Transcendental Meditation or TM.

A personal trainer learns to weigh risk versus benefit when creating an exercise routine. This mindset helps me to truly appreciate all that meditation has to offer. A study done by the Medical College of Georgia found that meditation can help you maintain a healthy heart.

In addition, the National Institutes of Health (NIH) now recommends meditation as part of the first line of treatment for high blood pressure. It has been used for thousands of years to treat chronic pain, drug addiction and possibly the biggest killer, stress itself. As far as I know there are no negatives.

Meditation and the Brain

Many people realize that regular meditation has a positive effect on them emotionally but does it actually change your brain physically? According to a study published in the journal *NeuroReport* the answer is yes. Led by Dr. Sara Lazar, the study revealed that parts of the cerebral cortex, the brain's outer layer, were thicker in those who regularly meditated. This region, the so-called grey matter, is responsible for starting and stopping all voluntary movements. These findings were reached through the use of MRIs.

Meditation and the Cardiovascular System

In May 2005, *The American Journal of Cardiology* published the results of a study that showed meditation, or more specifically Transcendental Meditation, reduces death rates related to cardiovascular disease by 23 percent.

Meditation and the Immune System

A study of breast cancer patients conducted at Loyola University discovered a strong link between meditation and immune function. Professor Linda Janusek, who headed the investigation, found that alterations in brain chemistry that result from meditation lead to a strengthening of the immune system.

In another study, conducted at University Of Wisconsin-Madison, changes in both brain and immune function were found in those who meditate. Richard Davidson, Ph.D., identified increased activation in the left side of the brain's frontal region in those who received training. They also demonstrated a marked increase in the production of antibodies. A control group of similar size was used to validate the findings and failed to produce similar results.

Meditation and Insomnia: A Plus for the Sleep Deprived

While meditation can improve everyone's health and quality of life, it is especially important for the growing percentage of the population who are sleep deprived. According to the National Sleep Foundation, "About 63 percent of Americans get fewer than 6.9 hours of sleep per night on average, about one hour less per night than they did thirty years ago." It has been determined that regular meditation helps the body compensate for the lack of a good night's sleep.

What is Meditation?

But what is meditation? Patricia Monaghan, co-author of *Meditation-The Complete Guide*, defines it as, "Activities (or lack of activities!) that center the person in the moment, that free the mind from the continual rant of the inner dialogue, and that promote (although often rather slowly) a more peaceful and serene approach to life."

Transcendental Meditation (TM)

Transcendental Meditation, or TM, is a method of meditation that has been taught for thousands of years. Originated in India, TM is now popular in many countries throughout the world. This method has been a part of my daily routine for nearly two decades; I've found it extremely beneficial both physically and mentally.

The Method

The practice of TM is surprisingly simple. You are assigned a mantra, a sound without meaning that you are not to reveal to others. This carefully chosen sound possesses a vibratory quality that enhances the experience, and has no associations that might prove distracting. Choose a comfortable position then sit quietly with your eyes closed for about 30 seconds. Next, begin thinking the mantra and continue doing so for the next 20 minutes. If thoughts creep into your consciousness, neither pursue them nor fight them. Instead, simply allow them to drift back out of your mind. Afterwards, sit quietly for about three minutes before slowly opening your eyes. This simple method is to be performed twice daily; once shortly after waking, and again later in the day.

The Program

Learning TM requires a commitment of about two hours per day for four consecutive days. The instructor chooses a mantra specifically for the individual. All meditations are supervised and all questions are answered. The drawback to TM is the price: Currently $2500 in the US. They do, however, offer free introductory lectures so that you can learn more before deciding to take the plunge.

In addition to receiving training in how to meditate, the TM folks offer something called a "checking". During these periodic follow-ups, those who have completed the course can return for a supervised meditation, free of charge. This allows them to make sure that everything is being done correctly as well as ask any questions they might have. Advanced courses are also available.

For more info on TM visit their website at: www.tm.org

9

or call: 1-888-LearnTM.

You can also read *TM - Transcendental Meditation* by Robert Roth (Plume; Rev&Updtd edition, September 1, 1994)

The Relaxation Response

This is the name used by Herbert Benson, MD, president of the Mind Body Medical Institute, for a style of meditation that he developed in the 1960's while doing research at Harvard Medical School. It is similar to Transcendental Meditation but without the brief, traditional ceremonies that accompany the studying of TM. Rather than being assigned a mantra, the individual chooses their own word. The number "one" is a popular choice as is the word "Om". While many TM proponents insist that nothing can match its time tested results, those shown by this style of meditation have been quite good.

For more info on the Relaxation Response visit the Benson-Henry Institute for Mind Body Medicine's website at: www.mbmi.org. Once there, click on the tab titled programs and services.

You can also read *the Relaxation Response* by Herbert Benson, MD (HarperTorch; Reissue edition, August 1, 1976)

An Easy Way to Meditate

If you're in a position to take a course, I would recommend doing so. Nothing beats high level instruction from a competent teacher. If not, there is no cause for alarm. Here are some simple instructions that will enable you to meditate quite effectively.

First, close your eyes and sit quietly for about 30 seconds. Next, begin thinking a word that has as few associations for you as possible. Let the word pass through your mind for the next 15-20 minutes. If thoughts pop into your head, don't fight them, simply disregard them, returning to the word that is your anchor. After the necessary time has passed, stop thinking the word, and sit quietly for two to three minutes before slowly opening your eyes. After your eyes have opened, give yourself a minute before slowly rising and beginning your day. While there are other methods, the one I described is simple and has shown excellent results.

Other Methods

There are many methods of meditation, each valid in its own way. The most popular include, Zen Meditation, Christian Prayer Meditation and Breath Awareness Meditation. Information on these and many other methods can be found in the suggested reading section at the end of this chapter. Feel free to experiment until you find the one that is right for you.

Meditation Dos and Don'ts

While thinking during meditation can be counterproductive, putting some thought into planning the experience is a must. Below are some tips that can help you to get the most from meditation:

Dos:

*Sit Comfortably: Discomfort can distract you, thereby interfering with your meditation. A chair with comfortable armrests is ideal. A couch with a cushion under each arm can also work nicely. When sitting up in bed and meditating, simply rest your arms on your lap. Avoid positions that you do not have the flexibility to sit in comfortably.

*Choose Comfortable Clothing: Select clothes that will not restrict your breathing. It is also advisable to remove your shoes. For your morning meditation these factors shouldn't be a problem. As for your evening meditation, keep them in mind and do the best you can.

*Choose a Quiet Environment: This can be a challenge, especially for city folk who cannot always find a quiet place to meditate. Don't let noisy surroundings worry you. Even though quieter is better, you can still benefit greatly from meditation done under such conditions.

*Check Your Watch if Necessary: While this isn't something you should do too often while meditating, if wondering how long it's been is proving to be a distraction, then a quick time check can put your mind at ease.

Don'ts:

*Don't Lie Down: While it may feel comfortable it is *too* comfortable and can easily lead to your falling asleep at the meditative wheel.

*Don't Eat Right Before: One of the goals of meditation is to slow down your bodily processes and digestion tends to speed them up. It is best to wait at least an hour after eating before you meditate. An advantage of meditating first thing in the morning is that this will not be an issue.

*Don't Meditate to Music: While soothing New Age music might

11

seem to set the mood, it is best to create as few distractions as possible. As a result, both music and your sound machine are best left out of the experience.

*Don't Set a Timer: Concern over meditating for too long, and as a result being late for work, might make this a tempting option. However, you will begin to anticipate the timer, thus interfering with the meditative process.

*Don't Forget Those Last Few Minutes: Remember to wait at least two to three minutes after meditating before opening your eyes, then another before jumping up and moving on. Those who skip this "transition" period are likely to pay for it with a feeling of irritability throughout their day, the exact thing you meditate to avoid!

Suggested Reading

How to Meditate: A Practical Guide by Kathleen McDonald Wisdom Publications; Reprint edition (March 25, 1984)

Meditation As Medicine by Dharma Singh Khalsa, MD (Fireside, 2002)

Meditation For Dummies by Stephen Bodian (IDG Books Worldwide Inc., 1999)

Meditation-The Complete Guide by Patricia Monaghan and Eleanor G. Viereck (New World Library, 1999)

"We never know the worth of water till the well is dry."
-French Proverb

"[Water is] the only drink for a wise man."
-Henry David Thoreau

2 | 7:20 a.m. How Much Water Will You Drink?

You're refreshed from a good night's sleep and your morning meditation. Now it's time to down the first of what should be numerous glasses of water.

Why Water Is Important

Surpassed only by oxygen in its significance to us, water is required for the performance of virtually every essential biological function. Our bodies are over 50 percent water and the loss of as little as one to two percent of your body weight can sap your energy. Water flushes toxins out of your system and aids in the healing process. It acts as a trucker, transporting nutrients throughout your digestive system and works hand in hand with fiber in the elimination of waste products. Water also aids in the regulation of body temperature. As a result, humans deprived of water die in a matter of days. So how much water should you drink?

Recommended Intake

We lose about 2.5 liters of fluid each day through urination, sweating and breathing, as well as our intake of dehydrating substances including sodium and alcohol. Since most of us get about 20 percent of that back in the food we eat, drinking two liters a day should replenish lost fluids. A popular rule of thumb is that you should drink eight 8 oz.

DAILY WATER INTAKE

| SUNDAY |
| MONDAY |
| TUESDAY |
| WEDNESDAY |
| THURSDAY |
| FRIDAY |
| SATURDAY |

glasses of water per day. This not only provides you with roughly 64 ounces of fluid per day, it also makes it easy to accurately schedule and keep track of your daily water intake. For example, you could drink one glass every two hours starting at eight a.m. Refer to the chart on page 14. By copying, then placing it somewhere visible you can check off each glass of water as you drink it, making it simple to keep track of how much water you drink.

A New Theory

A new theory proposes that you can allow thirst to be your guide in determining water requirements. A report authored by the Institute of Medicine of the National Academies in February 2004, claimed that there is not enough evidence to establish water intake recommendations as a means to reduce the risks of chronic disease. Many dissenters claim that thirst is merely a symptom of an already existing problem. According to the American Council on Exercise (ACE), relying on thirst as an indicator during exercise would only lead an individual to replace between 50 to 75 percent of their lost fluids. Also keep in mind that thirst, like hunger, tends to lessen as we age, making it a poor indicator of fluid needs. When using this method, check the color of your urine frequently. Producing urine that is dark in color, or that gives off a strong odor, may be an indicator of inadequate fluid intake.

Other Factors

Water Intake During Exercise

Since approximately 75 percent of your muscle tissue is water, it is easy to understand how dehydration could negatively impact both your health and athletic performance. The recommendation of the American Council on Exercise (ACE), is to drink a minimum of three to six ounces of water every ten to fifteen minutes during exercise. It also recommends drinking eight ounces between twenty and thirty minutes before exercise as well as eight to ten ounces within the half hour after your workout has been completed.

Water Intake and Weight Loss

Some people fear that drinking more water will cause them to gain weight. Not only is this belief false, but the opposite is true. When you drink too little water your body goes into conservation mode, retaining water for when it is needed. So when trying to shed excess weight, adequate hydration is key.

Health Conditions That Might Effect Recommendations for Fluid Intake

There are several health conditions that require you to drastically limit fluid intake, either at certain times of day or in total. Others require you to carefully monitor water quality. These include:

Advanced Kidney Disease: With the onset of kidney disease, toxins are not removed from the body and begin to accumulate. During the next phase, as urination tapers off, you must compensate by drinking less fluids. As the disease progresses, maximum daily fluid intake is usually limited to one liter, due to the body's inability to remove excess fluids. Fortunately, dialysis can serve both purposes by removing toxins and excess fluids, but can only eliminate approximately one liter per hour. As a result, fluid restrictions are necessary.

Gastric Bypass Surgery: For the more than sixty million Americans who qualify as obese, this procedure is becoming increasingly popular. While individuals who have had gastric bypass surgery are required to drink a minimum of sixty four ounces of water per day, their fluid intake *during* a meal must be tightly controlled. They are directed not to drink anything 30 minutes prior to, during, or for 60 minutes after a meal. Anyone contemplating this procedure should note the results of a recent study. It found that a significant percentage of those individuals who have had gastric bypass surgery died within one year.

Diseases of the Immune System: People with compromised immune systems need to be extra cautious when choosing their water supply. According to the EPA, people with AIDS, those on chemotherapy, and those taking drugs to avoid the rejection of a transplanted organ are more susceptible to contaminants than the rest of the population. They recommend that those individuals consume high quality bottled water.

Sodium Restricted Diets: Drinking water contains sodium; the question is how much? For most of us this is not an issue. The level of sodium in most drinking water is at a level generally considered safe. For people on sodium restricted diets, however, more careful monitoring of those levels is necessary.

Tips to Increase Water Intake

Until you get in the habit, drinking more water may slip your mind. Below are several tips to help you increase water consumption.

*Keep an empty glass in a visible place. It will serve as a reminder to drink up before continuing your morning routine.

*Bring a bottle of water to work. This enables you to drink small amounts throughout the day. A bottle with the ounces clearly marked is also a great way to keep track of your consumption.

*Create a water intake chart, like the one on page 14, then check off each glass as you drink it.

Choosing the Source

According to Carol Sorgen, MA, "Approximately seven million people become sick and more than 1,000 die in the U.S. each year from bacteria in their drinking water." It is a truly alarming statistic that makes you think long and hard about the source of your drinking water.

Bottled Water

So from what source should you get your water? Making the right choice is not as easy as it sounds. In his book, *The 100 Simple Secrets of Healthy People*, David Niven, Ph.D., states, "When tested by an independent group, one-third of the most popular bottled water in California supermarkets failed to meet state water quality standards, and all of the samples—100 percent—failed to meet advertised claims of purity." He claims that 40 percent of the bottled water sold in America is in reality tap water, not such a bad thing when you consider that bottled water is actually less regulated than what comes out of our faucet. In spite of this information sales of bottled water across the nation have doubled in the past ten years. Standards for bottled water safety and purity are set by the Food and Drug Administration. For more information consult their website at: www.fda.gov.

Information can also be obtained from the International Bottled Water Association (IBWA.) Visit their website at: www.bottledwater.org.

Tap Water

Whether your tap water is safe to drink depends to a great extent on where you live. Years ago when New York City was drowning in bad press, a study revealed that the quality of its drinking water was the best in the nation. New York City tap water even became a novelty item, sold in gift shops around Times Square. Unfortunately, not every city can hold its head as high. A good first step in deciding if your tap water is safe to drink is to contact your municipal water supplier. They can send you an annual water quality report that will list the levels of contaminants in your area. This will not, however, account for those impurities specific to your home. As home plumbing deteriorates over time, trace amounts of lead can contaminate the water that passes through it. To find information specific to your home, contact a water testing laboratory certified by your state. Standards for the quality of tap water are set by the Environmental Protection Agency (EPA). For further information you can consult the EPA's website at: www.epa.gov.

Keep in mind that not everything the EPA says is reliable. In December 2006 Daniel Storms, a monitor of New York water supplies, was sentenced to two months probation. Storms' crime was falsifying entries on water quality. He was the second New York City employee convicted of the crime in just over one year.

Well Water

Today over 20 million Americans still drink well water. Although this sounds like the healthiest choice of all, be aware that the regulation of water quality in private wells is extremely limited. Water that starts out pure can pick up contaminants, both man-made and environmental, that could potentially go undetected. Those whose wells are shallow, located near the bottom of a hill, or are in areas where animals graze should be especially careful. As a result, if you get your water from a well, periodic testing by a state accredited lab is advisable.

Methods of Purification

There are numerous methods of water purification. Some are expensive, time consuming or require a great deal of equipment. These are used by large companies trying to win the lion's share of the lucrative bottled water market. Two more practical methods are listed below. They are inexpensive and available to everyone.

Water Filters

Water filters work by forcing liquid through a screen that removes impurities. These devices eliminate a wide range of contaminants including lead, radon and pesticides. Effective, cheap and readily available, filters are an excellent choice for home use in purifying tap water. It is important to remember that each filter has a lifespan and needs to be changed periodically in order to remain effective.

Water Purifiers

More sophisticated than a filter alone, these devices add a disinfectant during the filtration process that kills all types of disease-causing organisms. These systems are popular with campers.

Invisible Dangers

"... a billion-and-a-half people never get a clean glass of water."
—Former President Bill Clinton

So what is it that we are being protected against? The EPA sets standards for about 90 different contaminants that are found in drinking water. Below are some hidden perils that can cause the water you drink to do more harm than good.

Bacteria

Bacteria are one-celled organisms. Unlike minerals that build up over time, bacteria like E. coli or Clostridium botulinum, which causes botulism, can prove deadly far more quickly. We usually think of problems of this nature as something experienced only in the Third World or as the result of some far-fetched terrorist attack. This is not always the case. Dangerous levels of E. coli were found in the polluted flood waters of New Orleans in the wake of Hurricane Katrina.

You can't discuss bacteria in drinking water without a mention of that old nemesis, amoebic dysentery. Better known as Montezuma's Revenge, this tiny terror is found in drinking water throughout Mexico. While it is not likely to kill you, it has ruined the vacations of many travelers.

Fluoride

Added to drinking water to protect our teeth, low levels of this commonly found element can prove beneficial. Higher concentrations can cause illness including skeletal fluorosis, a serious bone disease. Excess fluoride can be effectively removed through either distillation or reverse osmosis.

Hard Water

Hard water contains a high concentration of minerals, in particular calcium and magnesium. Since neither is considered harmful when ingested in reasonable amounts, hard water is not considered a health hazard. In reality, it can provide an added source of both minerals for those whose diets provide less than the RDA. Still, since hard water leaves behind a film that many find unappealing and can often clog appliances, many find it less than desirable. The problem can be controlled through the use of an ion exchange water softening unit.

Lead, Sodium and Chlorine

The effects of drinking water too high in lead can be devastating and include damage to both the kidneys and nervous system. In children, ingesting excess lead can delay both their physical and mental development. Because of this, pipes and other plumbing fixtures made of lead have been illegal since 1998. The amount of lead viewed as acceptable in drinking water is 15 parts per billion.

High levels of sodium in drinking water can contribute to hypertension, though it is unlikely that enough will be present to pose a substantial health risk for the majority of the population. Sodium is also a dehydrating substance. As a result, the more sodium in your drinking water, the more water you will require to achieve and maintain optimal health. The level listed as safe by the EPA is 20 milligrams per liter and is viewed by many as too conservative. Still, since excess sodium in the diet is undesirable, the less of it in your water the better.

Unlike lead and sodium, chlorine in drinking water is of great benefit. Chlorination provides us with a cheap, effective supply of water that is safe to drink. However, levels that far exceed the EPA's recommendation can result in a variety of symptoms including stomach distress and irritation of the eyes and nose. According to Stig Regli, policy analyst with the EPA, the problem isn't so much the chlorine itself but how it interacts with other substances. According to Mr. Regli, "Chlorine reacts with normally occurring organic materials to form byproducts that can present a health risk." The amount of chlorine viewed as acceptable is four milligrams per liter. The danger posed by high concentrations of chlorine can be illustrated by the fact that gas containing 1,000 parts per million can be fatal after just a few deep breaths.

Parasites

These single-celled organisms can be harder to kill than either bacteria or viruses. There are many harmful parasitic organisms that can be contracted through drinking water. They include:

Cryptosporidium: Both young children and pregnant women are especially vulnerable; can prove fatal to those with weakened immune systems.

Giardia: Found throughout the world including the United States. This one celled organism can lead to both dehydration and weight loss. It is the most common non-bacterial cause of diarrhea in North America.

Pesticides

The chemicals that farmers use to protect their crops can sometimes end up in your water supply. It is estimated that over 14 million people routinely drink water contaminated with five major agricultural herbicides. High levels of pesticides can cause cancer, birth defects and damage your nervous system. The EPA monitors pesticide levels in your drinking water. The results of these tests can be obtained by contacting your local water company.

Viruses

A virus can be defined as a simple microorganism capable of causing an infectious disease. Smaller than bacteria, these tiny organisms can infect water supplies. They include:

Hepatitis A: A tiny virus of intestinal origin. It infects up to 200,000 Americans annually, making it the seventh most common among all infectious diseases. Once contracted, it attacks the liver and results in approximately 100 deaths per year in the United States.

Noroviruses: A class of viruses often contracted through drinking water. Infection is referred to by several names including viral gastroenteritis and the stomach flu. In most cases, the effects are neither serious nor long term, but can result in several days of illness that can lead to dehydration.

Water Bottles

Few things seem less dangerous than your favorite water bottle. Still, the bacteria that build up after repeated use can cause numerous health problems.

- I know of a woman who developed sores in her mouth that were highly resistant to treatment. Doctors eventually traced the cause to bacteria that had built up on her favorite water bottle.

- In October 2002, CBS News reported that bottles that are not properly disinfected can lead to serious stomach problems.

- Another alarming report was issued by the *Canadian Journal of Public Health*. It stated that samples taken from the water bottles of elementary school students in Calgary contained concentrations of bacteria that were dangerously high.

If you plan to keep using the same bottle make sure to wash it thoroughly in water hot enough to kill any germs that may have accumulated over time.

Be aware that the harmful agents discussed in this section are only a few of the ones that can pollute our drinking water. Safe water is the most essential element to us after air. Therefore, taking sensible precautions in regard to the water you drink is highly recommended.

Water Alternatives

Oxygenated Water

The proponents of this potion claim that it improves stamina and athletic performance as well as cutting recovery time. It is also said to improve mental clarity. Research has failed to support these assertions:

* In a study conducted at the University of Wisconsin-La Crosse, the results indicated that oxygenated water did not increase the blood's oxygen supply. They attributed any benefit to the placebo effect.

* In November 2003, the *Journal of the American Medical Association* reported this product to have no discernable advantage over tap water in regard to the enhancement of athletic performance.

Sports Drinks

Sports drinks, like anything else that claims to give you a chemically engineered "edge", have been popular for quite some time. There are pluses and minuses to sports drinks, some of which are listed below:

Advantages: Studies have shown that brands with between six and eight percent carbohydrates, replace fluids faster than plain water. They also contain electrolytes, which physically active people may find beneficial.

Disadvantages: There are many of these products on the market, making a variety of different claims. This makes it difficult to know what to believe. Some brands can be pricey and they add calories to your daily total. Studies have shown a link between sports drinks and irreversible dental erosion.

Conclusion

Most of the research I've seen on sports drinks shows them to be no better than water for most people with typical fitness goals. Only elite athletes who need to perform maximally in a competitive atmosphere will truly benefit from these products under most conditions. A great deal has been written about them, so doing some research is recommended. Also, read the label carefully so that you know what you're drinking.

Enhanced Water

If you're exposed to the media, these products are hard to avoid. They are enriched with vitamins, or other potentially beneficial substances, and are purported to be healthier to consume than plain water. Below are some of the good and bad points of these popular beverages:

Advantages: Supplies those in need with a substantial quantity of vitamins and minerals. The "trendiness" of these products often results in people drinking more water than they normally would.

Disadvantages: Supplies those *not* in need with the same vitamins and minerals. As we will see throughout this book, more is not necessarily better. Many brands also contain stimulants, the exact quantity of which is not always specified.

Conclusion

It is wise to read up on these products before buying them. See that your research comes from independent sources, not just from the manufacturer who has a vested interest in your continuing to purchase their product.

Recommendation

All available studies seem to indicate that filtering your water, whatever the source, is a sensible decision. Make sure the filter is in good working order and is changed as recommended by the manufacturer. Remember that barring unusual circumstances, such as those listed earlier in this chapter, no upper limits have been set for water consumption. So drink up!

Want More Info?

Below are helpful websites for those who want further information about the safety of their drinking water:

www.awwa.org - The American Water Works Association

www.bottledwater.org - The International Bottled Water Association

"...a rose by any other name would smell as sweet."
—From *Romeo and Juliet* by **William Shakespeare**

3 | 7:25 a.m.
Will You Try Aromatherapy?

Another great way to relieve stress that takes little time out of your busy day is aromatherapy, a form of alternative medicine that has been practiced in Europe for over two hundred years. Aromatherapy can be defined as the use of aromatic compounds, derived from plants, to improve one's emotional state and/or physical health. Your sense of smell is powerful and communicates a wealth of important information to your brain. An objectionable smell can make you physically sick in a matter of seconds. Isn't it logical that a pleasing one can do just as much to improve your health?

Rene-Maurice Gattefosse

In 1910, a French chemist by the name of Rene-Maurice Gattefosse was working at a cosmetics company when a small explosion left one of his hands badly burned. Looking for a source of relief, the chemist immersed the wound in the first thing that was available to him, a vat of lavender oil. The rapid healing of the burn and lack of any noticeable scar led Gattefosse to experiment further. In 1928, he wrote a book entitled, *Aromatherapie*, and is credited with coining the phrase, aromatherapy.

How Therapeutic is Aromatherapy?

Everyone enjoys a pleasant fragrance and there are benefits that come from those positive feelings. Many also believe that aromatherapy can be a valuable compliment to traditional medicine in its treatment of a wide variety of ailments.

- In the December 2005 issue of *Prevention Magazine*, Virginia lawyer Valerie Szabo, discusses how aromatherapy helped her overcome the stress that was ruining her health.

- In 2005, a study was conducted to determine the effect of scent on people's sleep patterns. The study, which involved 31 test subjects, found that the scent of lavender was effective in inducing sleep. The results were reported in the journal, *Chronobiology International*.

- In her book, *Aromatherapy For Dummies*, Kathi Keville explains how scent can be used to combat health problems ranging from dry hair to carpal tunnel syndrome.

In The Nose of the Beholder: Choosing a Scent

While much has been written about the potential benefits of different scents, one fact appears conclusive; what smells good to you makes you feel good. This is born out by research conducted at England's Warwick University that showed a person's preference for a scent was a key to them benefiting from it. The best course of action is trial and error. Eventually you will find which aromas you prefer. Personally I'm quite fond of vanilla, a popular scent with many men. For you it could just as easily be lavender or chamomile.

Ways to Use Aromatherapy

Perfuming a Room

Burners

There are many ways to enjoy what aromatherapy has to offer. A practical and time efficient method is to perfume a room. This is the term Christine Wildwood used in her book, *Aromatherapy Made Easy*, to describe the use of an oil burner/vaporizer or electric fragrancer to disperse the scent throughout the area. Many people find the traditional looking burners more esthetically pleasing, while the electric version has several settings, allowing you to vary the intensity of the fragrance. Other ways to perfume an area are listed below.

Incense

Another way to quickly perfume a room is by burning incense. These aromatic compounds come in stick, cone or granulated form and a wide variety of aromas. Incense is usually made from a combination of oils, gums, wood powders and aromatic herbs and is both pleasing to smell and safe to breathe.

Scented Candles

Scented candles offer an alternative to incense and have the added visual allure of the flame, which many find soothing. Caution should always be used when burning scented candles. Some of the chemicals used to create the pleasing fragrance may not be safe to breathe and open flames left unattended can prove to be a fire hazard.

Potpourri

This scented mix of dried herbs and flowers is extremely popular. Housed in a variety of attractive containers, potpourri is as pleasing to the eye as it is to the nose. Unscented potpourri is also available. This allows you to spray the container's contents with a scent of your choosing. A fixative, often orris root, should be added to unscented potpourri to facilitate absorption.

Flowers

Let us not forget this most basic form of aromatherapy, the one handed to us by Mother Nature herself. The smell of flowers growing in a field or those in a vase next to your bed can make all the difference between the right and the wrong start to the day ahead. Take time to smell the roses!

Personal Uses

Perfume/Cologne

Personal preference is a factor when choosing a perfume or cologne. What smells great on one person might smell quite differently on another, so body chemistry must also be considered. We wear these scents for the pleasure of others, not just ourselves, so before loading up on what is the newest, hippest and most expensive scent on the market make sure to sample it first.

Scented Eye Pillows

When placed over your eyes, these handy little inventions fill the air around you with a pleasing fragrance. They are ideal for those who enjoy the smell of lavender, though other scents are also used. A word of caution, make your first application brief. You want to find out if you are allergic or in any way sensitive to something before leaving it on your face for half an hour. You can then gradually lengthen your exposure until you are comfortable that you and your scented pillow are compatible.

Pendants

Why not combine the visual appeal of jewelry with the benefits of aromatherapy? Wear a locket around your neck, filled with scented oil. Throughout your busy day it will fill the air around you with a pleasing fragrance.

Other Options

There are numerous other aromatherapy products that have personal uses. These include scented massage oils, facial saunas and steam inhalations. For more on these and other aspects of aromatherapy see the recommended websites and suggested reading list at the end of this chapter.

A Word about Safety

Fire: When burning something in your home, whether a candle or a stick of incense, be careful not to ignite anything other than what you intended. Safety precautions are necessary in order to keep this pleasant experience from becoming a tragic one.

Allergies: People are allergic to many things including the scents given off by products listed in this section. No matter how sweet the smell it should be avoided if it makes you ill. Common sense would dictate keeping your initial exposure brief. Be aware of any discomfort and discontinue contact at the first sign of trouble.

Taking it on the Road

While aromatherapy is a great way to start or end your day, its use is by no means limited to the home. Many of us spend a great deal of time in our cars, often under stressful conditions. Several forms of aromatherapy are available to you during your commute; they include:

Car Diffusers: Simply add a few drops of scented oil to a small pad, then place it inside the diffuser. By plugging this device into your car's cigarette lighter, you can then dispense the scent throughout the vehicle.

Car Jewelry: Place a few drops of essential oil, a concentrated, distilled liquid made up of aromatic compounds, inside these decorative vases or tiny clay figures, then enjoy the scent.

Sprays: Essential oils are also available in tiny spray bottles. This allows you to spray the scent of your choosing throughout your vehicle whenever the mood strikes you.

Conclusion

Pleasant odors are soothing and therefore improve our state of mind. While a medical professional should be involved in the treatment of any serious health condition, aromatherapy may help *prevent* illness by relieving the stress that weakens our immune systems. Why not give it a try?

Suggested Reading

Aromatherapy Made Easy by Christine Wildwood (Thorsons, 1997)

Aromatherapy for Dummies by Kathi Kaville (For Dummies, September 15, 1999)

The Complete Book of Essential Oils and Aromatherapy by Valerie Ann Worwood (New World Library, September 1991)

Want More Info?

For more information on aromatherapy, the National Association for Holistic Aromatherapy has an excellent website. Visit them at: www. naha.org.

The American Herb Association is directed by author Kathi Kaville. Visit them at: www.ahaherb.com.

"Variety's the very spice of life, that gives it all its flavor."
—William Cowper

4 | 7:30 a.m.
Have You Revised
Your Wardrobe Lately?

For more years than I care to count, I dressed pretty much the same way. From the mid-seventies through the late eighties I worked as a musician, playing the drums in rock clubs several nights a week. Because of the environment in which I spent most of my time, I was a jeans and tee shirt kind of guy. For footwear it was mostly sneakers or cowboy boots. For formal occasions I tossed on a polo shirt and for clubbing, some custom-made leather pants. Time went by and I worked in other settings but far too often I held onto that look or one fairly similar.

Eventually I decided to try something different. I started wearing dress pants and dress shoes and found out it didn't hurt a bit. Have you had the same look forever? Do you dress the same exact way no matter where you're going or what you're doing? Maybe you have two looks, one for work and one for everything else.

Vary Your Look

There was a *Seinfeld* episode where a girl Jerry was dating always wore the same outfit. He was dying to find out if they were the same *exact* clothes or if she had many copies of them hanging in her closet. What that show pointed out is that if you wear the same or very similar clothes *all* the time people *will* notice. It may also stifle your creative energy. This doesn't mean you have to wear something crazy.

No Hawaiian shirts or big pink hats are necessary just to show how versatile you are, but a brown suit and penny loafers *every* day?

Are You Stuck In a Time Warp?

Do you remember the best time of your life? Was it college, or the freedom you experienced after moving from a small town to a big city? Many people fixate on their glory days and never want to leave them behind. This attitude, while understandable, leads them to dress the same way now that they did then. You may have been hot stuff back in the day; still, wearing clothes that are clearly out of style will not only fail to recapture your past glory, but might also make you look a little foolish. Remember that times change, and so should your wardrobe.

Dress Your Age-Or Close to it

Most people will do whatever they can to look younger. The reality is, dressing the way the kids do may not do you justice. According to fashion expert Mary Lou Andre, if you try to look younger, you may end up looking older. "As you advance in age, your fashion options will drop off," claims Ms. Andre. She recommends that more mature women forgo the short skirts and sleeveless tops in favor of more age appropriate fashions.

Tips for Attaining Your New Look

Change is never easy. When it comes to your clothes or hairstyle, leaving that comfort zone can be extra traumatic. Below are a few ideas that might help nudge you in the right direction.

Give Your Old Clothes Away: Sometimes the best way to make room for something new in your life, or closet, is to get rid of some of what's already there. Numerous charitable organizations are more than happy to take your old things, and in many cases, pick them up as well. By doing so, you will open up some space, help those less fortunate, and may also receive a generous tax deduction. You can then take that money and purchase some new duds. The organizations listed below are reputable and will be happy to help.

Salvation Army	(800)-958-7825
Viet Nam Veterans of America	(631)-582-0242
Goodwill Industries	(301) 530-6500
Your Local House of Worship	

Read a Fashion Magazine: When looking for either a change of pace or a full makeover, fashion magazines are a good, inexpensive way to get some new ideas. In general, women are more familiar with these publications than men are, but they can be a great resource for both sexes. Some are exclusive to fashion while others merely include a section on the topic. Below are some good choices for him and her:

FOR HIM:	FOR HER:
Cargo	*In Style*
Instinct	*Allure*
Esquire	*Vogue*
Details	*Elle*
G.Q.	*Marie Claire*
Maxim	*Naturally You* (Hair)

Be Observant: This can be entertaining and costs you nothing. Whether you are at work or in a social setting, look at what others are wearing. I'm not saying that you need to buy earth shoes because the guy next to you is wearing a pair, but observing the more fashionable folks around you can be a way to get some new ideas and, unlike a magazine, you can ask him or her where they do their shopping.

Hire a Fashion Consultant: It's possible that your current wardrobe is not only too limited, but unflattering as well. Not sure what to wear? Sometimes it pays to hire a pro. Fashion consultants are expert at choosing clothes that allow you to look and feel your best. They are now employed by many Fortune 500 companies to work with their busy executives.

Hire an Image Consultant: Perhaps you want a full makeover. Image consultants not only spruce up your wardrobe, but your hair and makeup as well. Not sure what glasses look good on you? These folks can help. While once hired mostly by women, shows like *Queer Eye for the Straight Guy* have made employing a fashion consultant more appealing to men.

Hire a Color Consultant: Not everyone looks good in every color or has an eye for which ones look best on them. This is why professionals are available to help us. Color consultants are experts at choosing which colors are right for you. If you realize that you're wearing clothes that don't do you justice, then you might be more flexible about trying something new.

Hire a Personal Shopper: Filled with exciting new wardrobe ideas but too busy to shop for yourself? Not filled with *any* ideas and desperate for help? Third trip to the mall this week and still can't get a salesperson to look your way? Whatever the reason, many people hate to shop. Enter the personal shopper. For a fee, they will free you of the burden and fill your closet with things that are new, exciting, and right for you. For those who want some input but prefer not to pay for the service, many department stores supply personal shoppers to their customers free of charge.

Suggested Reading

In addition to the magazines mentioned earlier, the following books should be helpful to both men and women seeking to vary their look:

Dressing the Man: Mastering the Art of Permanent Fashion by Alan Flusser (HarperCollins, October, 2002) (Men)

Off the Cuff: The Guy's Guide to Looking Good by Carson Kressley (Plume, Reprint edition July, 2005) (Men)

The Lucky Shopping Manual: Building and Improving Your Wardrobe Piece by Piece by Andrea Linett and Kim France (Gotham, November, 2003) (Women)

Nothing to Wear? : A Five-Step Cure for the Common Closet by Jesse Garza and Joe Lupo (Hudson Street Press, March, 2006) (Women)

The Pocket Stylist: Behind-the-Scenes Expertise from a Fashion Pro on Creating Your Own Look by Kendall Farr (Gotham, January, 2004) (Women)

Ready to Wear: An Expert's Guide to Choosing and Using Your Wardrobe by Mary Lou Andre (Perigee Trade; Perigee edition March, 2004) (Women)

Want More Info?

If you'd like help finding an image consultant, visit the website of the Association of Image Consultants International (AICI), located at: www.aici.org.

"Sit up straight and eat your vegetables."
—Half the mothers who ever lived

"Slump and you'll get your grandmother's hump."
—The other half

5 7:34 a.m. Will You Check Your Posture?

Back in the 1930s, Dizzy Dean was a pitcher for the Saint Louis Cardinals. During the 1937 All-Star Game he was struck on the foot by a batted ball. As a result, Dean changed his pitching motion, ruined his arm, and prematurely ended his brilliant career. How does getting hit in the foot ruin your arm? A pitcher pushes off with his leg, the source of much of his power. With an injured foot he was no longer able to initiate his normal pitching motion. This story illustrates the often neglected link between the positioning and movement of one part of your body and the effect it has on all the other parts. This is an important concept to grasp when trying to understand how posture effects your entire body, and as a result, your quality of life.

Posture and Lower Back Pain

It is estimated that 80 percent of the American population suffers from lower back pain. Many experts believe that poor posture is a primary contributor to the problem. By positioning yourself in a way that is less than optimal, undue pressure is often placed on areas where nature never intended it to be. An example would be slouching, where the tilting of the pelvis exerts compressive forces on the spine. By bringing your body into proper alignment, much of that pressure can be relieved.

Posture and Tension Headaches

Tension headaches are that annoying pressure around your head or neck, caused by a tightening of muscles in those areas. While they can be brought on by a number of factors including stress, hunger and overexertion, a common cause is neck strain that results from poor posture. Temporary relief can be achieved through the use of medication however, that treatment option is complicated by dependency concerns and potential side effects. A more holistic approach would be to correct the cause, thereby alleviating its symptoms. If you feel that your headache may be the result of postural distortions, try the following:

Don't Slouch: Sit and stand up straight. This may stop your shoulder and neck muscles from tightening up.

Take a Break and S-t-r-e-t-c-h: Working too long in the same position can cause this type of problem. Periodically, take a few minutes to stretch before resuming your normal activities.

Work in a Comfortable Position: Some people work in positions that are awkward. If you find yourself stooping down or hunching over for prolonged periods of time try bringing your work surface closer to you.

Proper Posture

Also known as neutral alignment, ideal posture while in a standing position is achieved when the ankles, knees, hips and shoulders are both even and parallel to the floor. Your chest should be up and your shoulders back. Both sides of the body should be a reflection of each other.

When in a seated position, it is important not to slump, (lower back), or hunch, (upper back, shoulders, neck). These bad habits are often work related, the result of long hours spent driving or seated in front of a computer. They lead to the shortening of certain muscles, resulting in their inflexibility. At the same time, other muscles become overstretched and weak.

Keep in mind that restoring proper posture is not as easy as it sounds. Your body may have conformed to its new "shape" and forcing it back into proper position can cause problems to occur elsewhere. Several methods can be employed to fix what has gone wrong. They include the Alexander Technique, chiropractic, massage and flexibility training (stretching), all of which will be detailed later in this book.

Posture Tip: Watch What You Carry

Many people transport most or all of what they carry on one side of their body. This is true for the packages in your arms, the briefcase in your hand or the purse hanging from your shoulder. While it may *feel* natural, this type of uneven weight distribution can easily throw your back out of alignment, and may also result in injuries to the shoulder or neck. To avoid this type of injury, you should always balance what you carry as evenly as possible.

Many men walk around with something the size of a small suitcase crammed into their back pocket. Continually sitting with one side of your body higher than the other can throw your back out of alignment. Go through your wallet regularly and pull out things that you don't really need. Also consider varying the pocket in which you keep your wallet.

The Alexander Technique

"Alexander established not only the beginnings of a far reaching science of the apparently involuntary movements we call reflexes, but a technique of correction and self-control which forms a substantial addition to our very slender resources in personal education."
— **George Bernard Shaw**

During the latter part of the nineteenth century, an Australian actor by the name of F.M. Alexander, developed a serious case of laryngitis, which threatened his career. Doctors were unable to help him and after much self-analysis he determined that the tension in his neck, caused by his poor posture, was responsible. By changing the way he moved as well as how he positioned himself, Alexander was able to alleviate the problem and once again return to the stage. As a result of this experience he developed The Alexander Technique, a way of adjusting posture and movement patterns in order to better handle the challenges of daily life.

Proponents believe that studying Alexander helps you in a variety of ways. "When someone has their full upright posture their digestion is better," says Joan Arnold, an Alexander instructor in New York City. Ms. Arnold also feels that studying this method can help you to maintain a more youthful appearance. To illustrate the point she told me of a beautiful young woman who was seen from across the street by a group of her friends. From a distance each of them thought that they were looking at a much older woman, because of the way she carried herself.

Theory

Proponents of the Alexander technique believe that children are born moving in a proper and sensible way. In more primitive times, we maintained these movement patterns throughout our lives and as a result were free of many of the ailments that plague us today such as lower back pain. The development of these maladies can be blamed in part on technology, which advances at a pace far beyond that of the human body. This concept is supported by the fact that even today in cultures whose lifestyle more closely emulates our ancestors, many of those conditions are rare or nonexistent.

According to Richard Brennan, an Alexander instructor in Ireland, the technique will teach you to be more in tune with the physical laws of our world. Brennan states, "You will learn how to move with gravity, instead of against it, thus achieving greater ease of movement, this will in turn affect your mental and emotional outlook on life; you will feel calmer and therefore have a greater control of your own life."

Basic Concepts

Alexander believed that the head and spine have a relationship that affects the entire body. He dubbed this relationship primary control. His most fundamental concept is that when the neck does not overwork, the head can balance lightly at the top of the spine.

Proponents also believe that we often work too hard at movements that should be nearly effortless. "You can do more by doing less," says Joan Arnold in explaining the Alexander concept. Richard Brennan agrees, stating that, "Many adults often hold four or five times more tension in their bodies than is really necessary." He claims that this tension is responsible for many of the ailments that we mistakenly blame on the aging process.

For those who have never experienced an Alexander session, it is a far more subtle experience than many holistic health disciplines. The role of the instructor is that of a guide as you unlearn the faulty movement patterns and poor body positioning that have negatively impacted your quality of life.

While it can take many years to learn what Alexander discovered, there are certain basic recommendations worth noting. Many teachers feel that at least thirty lessons are necessary to get a true feel for what it has to offer. Taking several lessons a week during the initial weeks is encouraged in order to help you retain what you are taught in those early lessons.

Components

Direction: A way of using visualization that is a key component of every Alexander lesson. This is a technique used by instructors to help students internalize what they are being taught.

- In his book *Body Learning*, Michael J. Gelb gave an example of a student being told to picture, "His head floating like a helium balloon."

- In a study done by psychologist, Alan Richardson one group of basketball players practiced shooting free throws for twenty minutes a day while another visualized doing so. Amazingly, the improvement in their performance after twenty days was almost identical.

Postural Analysis: This is part of every Alexander lesson. According to Joan Arnold, "Posture is a result of how people use their muscles when they move." Observing this movement is an integral part of what an Alexander instructor does. They then convey that information to the student, enabling them to use it to correct faulty movement patterns.

Hands On: A student's limbs are gently manipulated by the instructor in order to convey a message. It is a subtle, gentle way of adjusting their natural movement pattern into one with more ease and comfort.

Qualifications

When working with someone who is going to help you change the way you use your body, it is important to know that individual is qualified. When it comes to the Alexander Technique, the training required varies based on the program attended as well as the certifying body with whom it is recognized. Quality training programs include: The American Center for the Alexander Technique (ACAT), Alexander Technique School New England (ATSNE), Alexander Technique Institute of Los Angeles (ATI-LA) and The Constructive Teaching Centre, located in London. If an instructor has a certification other than those listed, you can check with the following two certifying bodies to see which programs they recognize:

The American Society for the Alexander Technique (AmSAT):
www.alexandertech.org.

Alexander Technique International (ATI), who can be reached at:
www.ati-net.com.

Alexander and Aging

Many people, instructors and students alike, believe that by using this efficient method of movement, many of the ravages of aging can be delayed. According to Missy Vinyard, director of the Alexander Technique Center New England, "Perhaps the greatest factor in maintaining our quality of life as we age is the simple ability to move easily and without pain, so that we can accomplish the everyday tasks of living with pleasure and skill." Ms. Vinyard believes that by using Alexander's teachings to overcome excess tension and poor posture, we can avoid developing a wide variety of age related ailments including spinal curvature and fracture, arthritis and musculoskeletal injuries.

Summary

It is fair to say that Alexander can help most everyone on some level. This is true for individuals seeking to overcome pain that has come from poor posture or the misuse of certain muscles. It is also helpful to an athlete looking to enhance their performance or a performer looking to improve their poise on stage.

Suggested Reading

Body Learning: An Introduction to the Alexander Technique by Michael J. Gelb (Owl Books, 2nd edition, January 15, 1996)

The Alexander Technique Manual by Richard Brennan (Gardners Books, January 31, 2005)

Indirect Procedures: A Musician's Guide to the Alexander Technique by Pedro de Alcantara (Oxford University Press, April 24, 1997)

"Cleanliness is indeed next to godliness."
— **John Wesley**

6 7:40 a.m.
How Often Will You Wash Your Hands?

Some tiny life forms that we pay little attention to can make us very sick. I'm referring to germs picked up from surfaces that we touch. Whether it is the railing in the subway, the doorknob of your office or your best friend's hand, the germs you come in contact with can easily lead to a wide variety of illnesses. Let's look at the problem and some solutions.

Handshaking

In Western culture, there is no polite way around this standard method of greeting others. Still, some of us have been known to take it to extremes. On New Year's Day 1907, President Theodore Roosevelt was said to have set a record by shaking exactly 8,150 hands. While being friendly is commendable, there are risks to all that glad-handing. It is estimated that personal contact accounts for as much as 80 percent of all infectious diseases and handshaking is one of the main culprits. This is partly because many of us don't wash our hands as often as we should. In a study conducted by Wirthlin Worldwide, 22 percent of travelers visiting airport bathrooms failed to wash their hands before exiting. Assuming people were no tidier in Roosevelt's time, that means that on that fateful day in 1907 our president shook approximately 1,793 unwashed hands. How many hands did YOU shake yesterday?

Solutions

Washing Your Hands

There are over 200 cold-causing viruses living on surfaces all around us. Good old-fashioned hand washing is still the best method when trying to wipe out whatever germs you have picked up along the way. Make sure to use warm running water and plenty of soap. Rub your hands together vigorously for a minimum of 15 to 20 seconds. Wash your entire hand, front and back as well as your wrist. One place where germs often hide is under your nails so be sure to clean there as well.

Soap

Though soap-like products have been is use for over 4000 years, true soap was developed by the Phoenicians, around 600B.C. They combined goat fat, water and ash into a product similar to the one we use today. Soap works by reducing the skin's surface tension thereby attracting dirt and oil away from its surface.

Antibacterial Soap

Many types of bacteria can make you sick, so killing these tiny organisms may seem like a good idea. The problem is that bacteria are adaptable. Since many of these products use synthetic chemicals to perform their dirty work, the creatures they are killing may eventually evolve into a heartier strain that is resistant to those chemical agents. These new "super germs" could present health concerns that are far more serious than those posed by their predecessors. Also, keep in mind that while some bacteria are healthy, antibacterial soaps kill indiscriminately. Because of this, regular use of antibacterial soaps is not recommended.

Hand Sanitizers

There are times when you're not near a sink, so this convenient invention can help. You can buy a box of one hundred sanitizing hand wipes for a couple of dollars, or opt for the gel form with products like Purell. In order to be effective, brands that are alcohol based should contain 60-90 percent of the active ingredient. Be careful not to overuse these products. They tend to dry your skin which may cause it to crack, allowing bacteria to enter. Some products contain vitamins A and E as well as aloe to help rejuvenate your skin.

When to Wash

Always wash your hands before:

*Leaving the Gym: In a busy gym, exercise equipment is touched by hundreds of people a day, making it the perfect breeding ground for germs.

*Eating: Germs can easily be transferred from your hands to your mouth. In spite of this, it is estimated that one out of every three Americans doesn't wash their hands before eating. Make sure to wash your hands often and do so thoroughly before every meal. Hand washing is also advisable before touching your mouth, nose or eyes.

*Preparing Food: This is important since it involves not only your health but the health of those you love. The tasty meal you are about to prepare can easily become more harmful than healthful if you allow germs that you've picked up to climb on board. Be aware that many foods contain bacteria—salmonella in chicken, E. coli in vegetables—so be sure to wash your hands thoroughly before touching other food. Be extra vigilant about hand hygiene if you stop preparing a meal to pet the dog or use the bathroom.

Always wash your hands after:

*Using the Bathroom: Many illnesses can be prevented by practicing good hygiene. Common parasites such as cryptosporidium and giardia can be washed away with soap and water before they can become a threat. Another option, cover faucets and doorknobs with a paper towel before handling them.

*Using Shared Office Equipment: Copy machines and fax machines are essential tools for any busy office. They are also home to an impressive collection of germs. Numerous studies have found that telephones which are not regularly disinfected are dirtier than your bathroom floor.

*Reading in Waiting Rooms: The periodicals in a doctor's office are handled by dozens of people, and unless he's a dentist they are probably sick. While the magazines left in conference rooms and office waiting areas might fare better, it is unlikely that the hands they pass through are germ free.

*Holding on to Handrails: In a crowded store or train station, thousands of people a day will touch the same surfaces. Some of the most commonly handled are handrails. Escalator handrails are considered one of the dirtiest of all public surfaces.

*Pushing a Shopping Cart: In a busy supermarket, hundreds of people have handled that cart before you. Because of this, it is wise to wash your hands before eating the food you just purchased.

*Handling Money: Few things are as dirty as money. Both bills and coins have passed through countless hands before reaching yours. If you dine in a place where you pay before you eat remember to give your hands a once over before enjoying your meal. Keep a sanitizing hand wipe available for those occasions when a bathroom is not available.

Drying Your Hands

Wet hands transfer germs more easily than dry ones. As a result, how you dry your hands is just as important as how you wash them. With single-use paper towels, use one to remove most of the moisture, then another to dry them thoroughly. Recommended drying time is fifteen to twenty seconds. Many restrooms offer only air dryers. When using these machines, rub your hands together while rotating them. Recommended drying time is between thirty and forty-five seconds. Cloth towels, especially those that have been used by other people, are a potential breeding ground for germs. They should be avoided whenever possible.

Interesting Fact to Ponder
Less than two hundred years ago it was not customary for doctors to wash their hands before seeing patients. This practice, unthinkable today, continued until the mid-1800s. It was then that Dr. Semmelweis, an Austrian physician, pioneered the concept of good medical hygiene, much to the dismay of his superiors. Their resistance to his ideas persisted until he was able to use his sanitary principles to quell an epidemic of puerperal fever that was rampant in an Austrian hospital.

Even today, cleanliness within the medical community remains a concern. In the June 1995 issue of the *Journal of Hospital Infection*, some disturbing findings were published. The research conducted at Georgetown University stated that sporadic, ineffective hand washing was still the norm among all types of staff and in all health care settings. This is even more frightening when you consider that healthcare related infections are responsible for the death of approximately 90,000 Americans annually.

Suggested Reading

The Secret Life of Germs by Philip M. Tierno, Jr., Ph.D., (Atria; Reprint edition, January 1, 2004)

Want More Info?

If you'd like more information on this topic there is a very informative website run by The Soap and Detergent Association (SDA). Visit them at: www.cleaning101.com.

"For a long and healthy life, you should breakfast like a king, lunch like a prince and dine like a pauper."
—**Adelle Davis**

7:45 a.m.
Will You Eat Breakfast?

For years, I watched my mother enjoy her customary breakfast of coffee and cigarettes. I believe it was that behavior, combined with her lack of exercise that led to her frailty and poor health. Breakfast is the meal most often skipped, but also the most important. Your body can only store glycogen, (the storage form of carbohydrates), for about twelve hours. After that, it starts breaking down muscle and using it for fuel. This fact should be passed along to the approximately one in five Americans who regularly skip this opportunity to start their day off right.

Skipping Breakfast and Weight Loss

Skipping breakfast slows the metabolism, making it more difficult to lose weight. In addition, studies have shown that people who pass up their morning meal tend to overcompensate by eating extra calories over the course of the day. Remember that many breakfast foods are high in fiber, a key factor in feeling full.

Breakfast and Diabetes

Whole grains, common in many quality breakfast foods, are high in chromium and vitamin B6, two key weapons in the fight against diabetes. The high fiber content of these foods also increases satiety, thereby decreasing overeating, often a contributing factor in the development of type II diabetes.

Breakfast and Hypoglycemia

Hypoglycemia is a condition that occurs when the blood contains too little sugar. Delaying breakfast for those with hypoglycemia can be a particularly bad choice, a situation made worse if the last thing eaten was a snack high in simple sugar. The high concentration of sugar suddenly dumped into the hypoglycemic's blood stream shortly before bed, can lead to an overreaction by their system leading to a dangerous drop in sugar levels. The result of this is often dizziness or a nasty headache.

Breakfast and Memory

Numerous studies have shown a connection between eating a balanced breakfast and mental function, particularly memory. In a study done by Massachusetts General Hospital in Boston, using one hundred inner-city children as subjects, a correlation was found between eating breakfast and higher academic and social functioning.

In another study performed by Tufts University, children who ate breakfast were found to be higher performing. Additional gains were found among those who ate higher quality breakfast foods.

Breakfast and Celiac Disease

Celiac disease is a condition typified by an inflammatory response to gluten, a protein found in wheat, barley, and rye. Symptoms include, but are not limited to, abdominal pain, fatigue, anemia and a feeling of weakness. If ignored, celiac disease can lead to serious nutritional deficiencies. Since many breakfast foods such as cereals and muffins are high in gluten, it is essential that those suffering from this illness are extremely careful about their diets. More information about celiac disease can be found on the following websites:

www.celiac.com

www.glutenfree.com

www.csaceliacs.org

The Proper Nutrient Breakdown

If I want to choose a stock to invest in, I listen to the opinions of ten highly respected experts and if most of them agree that the stock is a good choice, then it probably is. I treat nutrition the same way. While there are all kinds of crazy diets out there, the real experts including the

American College of Sports Medicine (ACSM) and the US Department of Agriculture (USDA) make recommendations that are similar. Those recommendations include a diet consisting of approximately 50-60 percent carbohydrates, about 15-20 percent protein and about 20-30 percent fat. A high percentage of the carbohydrates should come from fruits, vegetables and whole grains. Saturated fats should be kept to a minimum. It is also suggested that you choose foods that are as unprocessed as possible. Below are some good choices for breakfast. Recommendations for other meals will be given later in the book.

The Low-Carb Conspiracy

You can't discuss nutrition without touching on this very controversial subject. In spite of the popular low-carb fad, carbohydrates are your body's preferred fuel source and should make up the bulk of your diet. Here's why:

Low-carb diets are by nature high in fat and low in fiber, which increases your risk of both cancer and heart disease.

When you take in fats, your liver must produce bile to help break them down. The more fat you consume the more bile you produce and store in your gallbladder. Bile leaves behind minerals that help to form gallstones.

If you take in too few carbs, your body must convert protein to carbohydrates through a process called gluconeogenesis. This produces ammonia, which is a poison. Your liver must then convert ammonia to urea and ship it to your kidneys to be excreted. Therefore, such a diet makes both your liver and kidneys work overtime.

Too much protein in your diet can turn your blood acidic. This forces your body to leech calcium from your bones in order to return your blood's PH to acceptable levels. This leads to a loss of bone mass which can be devastating in later years.

A low-carb diet leads to dehydration, the source of your initial weight loss. This belief is echoed by James Dillard, MD, assistant clinical professor at Columbia University College of Physicians and Surgeons in New York City. "... restricting carbohydrates causes you to lose weight -- but you'll gain it all back," says Dillard. "You're losing water in your system."

It Can't Be Bad, It's Organic

Organic foods are those grown without the use of pesticides or artificial fertilizers. According to U.S. Department of Agriculture regulations, food must contain at least 95 percent organically produced ingredients in order to be labeled organic. These products make up the fastest growing segment of the market, with 2005 sales topping $13.8 billion in the U.S. alone. Those who eat these foods have lower levels of pesticides in their bodies, and the rich soil in which they are grown result in higher levels of certain minerals. The way organic food is produced is also healthier for the environment. Be aware that the organic label is not a guarantee that food is healthier to eat and that certain foods, such as salmon, can be labeled organic even though the USDA organic standard does not apply to fish.

Be wary of the term "all natural". Remember that poison ivy is all natural and so is fertilizer. This doesn't mean that either is healthy or a good addition to your diet. Be aware that there are just as many "all natural" substances that can harm or even kill you as there are artificial ones. Also, be aware that while government standards exist for what can be labeled organic, the term "all natural" is as yet unregulated.

Some Good Breakfast Choices

Since we're making breakfast part of your daily routine, let's do so in a way that is both healthy and satisfying. Remember that healthy does not have to mean complicated. Below is a list of some good breakfast choices.

A bowl of whole grain cereal with soymilk and a handful of fresh fruit: Choose brands that are high in fiber, at least five grams per serving. Those worth considering include Go Lean and Mueslix. They contain a good balance of vitamins and minerals along with plenty of fiber. As for milk, think soy! It is believed that soy helps prevent the buildup of plaque on the walls of your arteries, thereby decreasing the likelihood of a heart attack or stroke. Soy may also reduce your risk of developing osteoporosis as well as certain cancers. If you don't have a taste for soy, skim milk is also a good choice. If neither is to your liking, then milk with one percent fat is also acceptable. As for fruit, blueberries are a great choice, as are strawberries or raspberries.

A low fat yogurt with some fresh fruit: Combines a great overall balance of protein, fat and carbohydrates. Studies have shown that people who eat yogurt regularly, have an easier time losing and keeping weight off, possibly due to its high calcium content. The active cultures contained in yogurt help to prevent stomach infections by encouraging healthy bacteria to multiply. The added fruit is loaded with cancer-fighting antioxidants.

A bowl of oatmeal: Oatmeal has been shown to help lower both blood pressure and levels of low-density lipoproteins (LDL.) High levels of LDL have been linked to an increased risk of heart disease. Add a handful of raisins, some walnuts or a spoonful of peanut butter for additional benefit. Top with cinnamon.

A poached egg on a whole wheat bagel: This provides a good combination of protein, fiber and complex carbohydrates.

Eggs and salsa in a whole wheat tortilla with black beans and low fat cottage cheese: This supplies a great combination of nutrients with the tangy taste that many people crave.

Remember that one of the keys to healthy eating is to eat *slowly*. It's a natural tendency for many of us to gulp our food down like someone is trying to take it away from us. This is even more common during breakfast when we're often in a hurry to get the day started. Playing some relaxing music with a slow tempo has been shown to help. In any event, whether you plan a musical breakfast or not, take a deep breath, and slow down!

Food Bars

This is the breakfast of choice for many who consider their mornings far too hectic to stop, smell the roses and eat properly. Unfortunately, much of their popularity can be attributed to convenience and lots of marketing rather than their value as a true breakfast substitute. Food bars aren't necessarily *bad,* but they are not the same as eating a balanced breakfast, and shouldn't be used as such on a consistent basis. But if it's a food bar you must have, then it pays to choose wisely.

Clif Bar: On those occasions when you choose to take the quick and easy way out, a Clif Bar is a good way to go. Unlike many of its competitors, which are little more than glorified candy bars, Clif Bars have a nice balance of nutrients including a substantial amount of fiber, usually around five grams per bar, and come in a variety of flavors.

Meal Replacement Drinks

Drinking your breakfast is another option. These time savers are often used by dieters in place of meals. Are they a good choice? So far the reviews are mixed. According to nutritionist Dr. Jane Pentz, only 15 percent of Americans eat the recommended amount of fruits and vegetables. She feels that dependency on both food bars and meal replacement drinks are partly to blame. In contrast, Australian researchers found that meal replacements can be as effective as many diet programs in facilitating weight loss. Those findings, published in the *Journal of Nutrition,* offer hope to those looking to drink those extra pounds away. Should you decide to substitute a meal replacement for a balanced breakfast, make sure that you choose wisely. The nutrient breakdown should be similar to that in the meal it is replacing, with a healthy mix of protein, fat and carbohydrates. Remember to read the label to make sure you are not just drinking something that tastes good but provides little benefit.

Condiments: The Real Problem

I have always felt that the problem with the average American diet is not so much what we eat as it is what we put on what we eat. This is true for every meal, breakfast included. Here are some condiments to avoid.

Butter and Margarine: Too many people drown a perfectly good muffin in this stuff. The saturated fat and cholesterol in butter and the trans fatty acids and chemicals in margarine are killers. Keep them to a minimum if you use them at all.

Salt: Sodium intake contributes to high blood pressure, particularly as we age. It is a factor in hardening of the arteries and causes you to retain water. It can also lead to fluid buildup in your lungs which makes breathing more difficult.

Sugar: Large quantities of refined sugar raise your levels of both blood sugar and stress hormones, two factors in the development of type II diabetes. Sugar also prematurely ages cells and is a known carcinogen. These facts are scary when you consider that the average American diet contains about one hundred fifty pounds of refined sugar per year.

Some Better Choices

Hummus: Dresses up a whole wheat pita nicely without the fat and sugar content of many other condiments.

Flaxseed Meal: When sprinkled on cereal or salad, this nut flavored, heart-friendly seed increases the health value of food rather than decreasing it. Flaxseeds are the most concentrated source of lignans, chemical compounds that have demonstrated antioxidant properties.

Benecol: A great replacement for butter or margarine. Benecol has been shown to help lower cholesterol levels.

Cinnamon: A great topping for cereal or oatmeal. Cinnamon has shown the ability to help regulate blood sugar. Moderate intake may also have a beneficial effect on cholesterol levels.

Fasting

Now that we've discussed what you *should* eat let us examine fasting, the concept of not only skipping breakfast but all the meals of the day and possibly several days to come. Fasting can be defined as willingly abstaining from food and possibly drink, for a period of time. It is an idea embraced by many cultures throughout history. Today, fasting is practiced by many holistic health enthusiasts. The question remains: Is it a healthy choice? Opinions are mixed.

According to Fasting Center International (www.fasting.com), the fasting process removes the 5-10 lbs. of toxic chemicals which are locked into the average adult's cell, tissue and organ storage areas. A conflicting opinion is offered by Dr. Jane Pentz who states:

> "Catabolism occurs when fasting. Precious muscle is used for energy. I know the alternative medicine world recommends fasting as a way of cleansing the body. However, we cannot cleanse our bodies through fasting since, unlike cars, our bodies are never "turned off" (until death). The only way to cleanse the body is through eating healthy foods with lots of antioxidants (whole grains, fruits, veggies, etc.)"

Keep in mind that not eating doesn't mean not drinking. Most fasting regimens include liberal amounts of water, juice or other liquids. The purpose of this fluid intake is to both enhance the benefits and mitigate the consequences of not eating for a period of time.

Food Allergies

One thing to consider when choosing the components of any meal is the potential harm produced by a food allergy. This occurs when your immune system mistakenly identifies a harmless substance as harmful and stages an unnecessary and unwelcome counterattack. These reactions, which occur in approximately 1 in 50 adults, are unpleasant and in rare cases can be serious or even fatal. A sudden, severe allergic reaction can result in a condition called anaphylaxis which requires immediate medical attention.

In order to protect the public from this danger, the Food Allergen Labeling and Consumer Protection Act of 2004 (FALCPA) was passed. It requires manufacturers to list clearly on the product's label, the presence of protein derived from any of the eight ingredients most likely to cause an allergic reaction. For more information on food allergies visit: www.foodallergy.org.

Suggested Reading

So What Can I Eat?!: How to Make Sense of the New Dietary Guidelines for Americans and Make Them Your Own by Elisa Zied (Wiley, February 2006)

What to Eat by Marion Nestle (North Point Press, May 2, 2006)

Consider subscribing to the *Nutrition Action Healthletter*. It offers quality information on a variety of nutritional topics. You can find it at:www.cspinet.org/nah/index.htm.

Want More Info?

The United States Department of Agriculture (USDA) has established a site that discusses the new food pyramid. It is filled with useful information. You can find it at: www.mypyramid.gov.

"Better safe than sorry."
—Irish Novelist Samuel Lover

8 | 7:45 a.m. Will You Take a Multivitamin?

A multivitamin is good low calorie nutrition. Taken with a balanced breakfast it will start your day off right. Many people feel that eating properly should be enough. While that's good in theory, few of us have diets that mirror the food pyramid. For those individuals who do, a well publicized study raises additional concerns. It was reported by Donald Davis, a University of Texas biochemist, that the fruits and vegetables we consume have less vitamins and minerals than they once did. Adding a multivitamin is one of the best and cheapest insurance policies you will ever take out.

A word of caution: The substances that a good multivitamin contains have been carefully balanced. Taken regularly they can improve both your health and quality of life. Taking mega doses of individual vitamins is another story entirely. Unusually high concentrations of fat soluble vitamins (A, D, E, and K), can be toxic. Dosages of vitamin A that are in excess of 10,000 IU per day have been linked to birth defects and daily intake of vitamin E that exceeds 800 IU has been known to depress the immune system.

Most people believe that you can't take too much of a water soluble vitamin. This is because the excess is excreted in the urine. However, if your body gets accustomed to an extremely high level of a water soluble vitamin, and the dosage is suddenly cut to a level more in line with the RDA, symptoms of deficiency can show up. This has been known to happen with vitamin C and can lead to an illness called rebound scurvy, which produces scurvy-like symptoms even though no deficiency exists.

An additional word of caution: Vitamins are *not* food. What they do is help your food to work more efficiently. A vitamin is a coenzyme. It helps enzymes perform their normal functions. Therefore taking a vitamin *instead* of breakfast is a very poor choice, not to mention the waste of a perfectly good vitamin.

Below is a list of vitamins and minerals commonly found in most multivitamins, along with some of their key functions in preserving your youth and health. Make sure they are included in the brand you choose.

Vitamins

Vitamin A: A potent antioxidant necessary for proper bone growth. Deficiency leads to vision problems including night blindness.

Vitamin C: A potent antioxidant critical to the production of collagen. It is also necessary for the production of certain hormones.

Vitamin D: Essential for the maintenance of a strong skeletal structure. It improves your body's ability to utilize calcium and regulates the level of phosphorous that is present in the bloodstream. This key nutrient may be the vitamin most deficient in the average American diet.

Vitamin E: A potent antioxidant that lowers the risk of heart disease. This essential nutrient may also reduce the risk of developing other age related diseases including both Alzheimer's and Parkinson's.

Vitamin K: A potent antioxidant that is crucial to blood's ability to clot. Vitamin K aids in calcium absorption and may play a role in the prevention of both heart disease and osteoporosis.

Thiamin (B1): Required by the body in order to metabolize carbohydrates. Thiamin also keeps the nervous system healthy. During the 19th century, the importance of thiamin was made crystal clear. White rice was substituted for brown in several Far Eastern countries, depriving the population of its primary source of thiamin. An outbreak of beriberi, a disease resulting from a thiamin deficiency, ensued.

Riboflavin (B2): Aids in the growth and repair of tissue. Those who exercise require more riboflavin due to heightened usage. Deficiency leads to an inability to utilize folic acid, a key nutrient in the fight against cancer. There is a possible connection between riboflavin deficiency and cataracts, an age-related eye condition which results in impaired vision.

Niacin (B3): Has shown the ability to reduce cholesterol levels. There is evidence that adequate intake of niacin cuts the risk of developing Alzheimer's disease by as much as 70 percent.

Vitamin B6: There is strong evidence that B6 reduces the risk of heart disease. It fights diabetes by increasing insulin sensitivity. It may also help to reduce skin cancer risk. There appears to be a connection between B6 deficiency and asthma.

Vitamin B12: Helps cells to reproduce and keeps nerve tissue healthy; can be helpful in fighting depression. A deficiency can result from a dangerous condition called pernicious anemia. Since our ability to absorb B12 may decrease with age, maintaining an adequate supply is crucial.

Folic acid: Adequate intake may reduce your risk of cancer, depression and diminished mental capacity. It also helps to reduce your blood's level of homocysteine, a type of amino acid that has been linked to a higher risk of heart attacks and strokes.

Biotin: Plays a role in the metabolism of glucose. Studies have found lower biotin levels in those suffering from type II diabetes. Biotin is required for the production of energy and certain enzymes.

Pantothenic Acid: Aids in the breakdown and utilization of protein, fats and carbohydrates. It also helps the brain and nervous system to communicate.

Minerals

Minerals are broken down into two categories, macro and trace depending on whether the body needs larger or smaller daily dose in order to maintain optimal health.

Macro: Daily requirements are between 100 mg and 1 gm

Calcium: The most abundant mineral in the human body. Calcium has the ability to build bone mass which helps to fight osteoporosis. Calcium also helps blood to clot, and regulates your heartbeat as well as proper functioning of your muscles and nerves.

Magnesium: Essential for metabolism of both carbohydrates and fats.

Deficiency can lead to a higher risk of both osteoporosis and anemia. Magnesium works together with calcium to perform many essential bodily functions.

Potassium: A key factor in the battle against both heart disease and diabetes. Potassium controls the functioning of all muscles including the heart as well as the release of insulin from the pancreas. Your ratio of sodium to potassium is crucial to maintaining each cell's internal and external fluid balance, so the more sodium you consume the more potassium you need.

Trace: Daily requirement is less than 100mg

Zinc: Hailed as an immune booster, this mineral is far more than that. Zinc is the light switch that flips on a wide variety of bodily functions. Zinc helps cells multiply and tissues regenerate. It regulates insulin metabolism and proper sexual function. Zinc has been shown to protect against macular degeneration, an age-related eye condition that often leads to blindness. Zinc restores proper functioning to the thymus gland, which tends to lose function with age. It has also been shown to have antioxidant properties. Deficiency can lead to an increased risk of osteoporosis.

Iodine: Deficiency can lead to an increased risk of hypothyroidism and brain damage.

Selenium: This potent antioxidant is a key weapon in the fight against prostate cancer, the second most common form of cancer found in men. Selenium may reduce the risk of developing age-related conditions such as heart disease and arthritis.

Copper: A lack of copper is a prime contributor to heart disease, anemia and diseases of the central nervous system. A deficiency also causes bones to fracture more easily.

Manganese: Plays a role in the formation of bone and connective tissue. Deficiency can lead to an increased risk of both osteoporosis and arteriosclerosis.

Chromium: Studies have linked low levels of chromium to diabetes. This is partially because the mineral increases one's sensitivity to insulin.

Molybdenum: A cofactor for three enzymes, the functions of which are essential to human life. This mineral helps break down toxins so that they can be removed from the body and also helps to prevent tooth decay. Deficiency may lead to impotence in older males.

Iron: Insufficient iron in the blood can lead to lethargy. Iron is needed for the production of amino acids, the building blocks of protein. Deficiency can eventually lead to anemia, a condition where the body's tissues become starved for oxygen. Other maladies related to insufficient iron intake include impaired mental development and an increased risk of infections and certain types of cancer.

To learn more about how the vitamins and minerals in our diet affect our health, there is an excellent website run by the Linus Pauling Institute's Micronutrient Information Center. Visit them at: lpi.oregonstate.edu/infocenter

Choosing a Brand

Choosing the right supplement has never been easy but an act passed in 1994 made it even more difficult. Since the passage of the Dietary Supplement Health and Education Act (DSHEA), supplements have been deregulated and no longer require approval from the FDA or any other certifying body. Fortunately for consumers there are several trustworthy organizations that evaluate vitamins that are submitted to them on a voluntary basis. Upon review, if the vitamin or supplement is found to be satisfactory, it is given a seal of approval by that organization.

Below are the websites of three such institutions. By checking with them, you can feel more confident that you are getting safety and value for your money. They are:

U.S. Pharmacopeia: www.usp.org

ConsumerLab: www.consumerlab.com

NSF International: www.nsf.org

How to Maintain Potency

Vitamins lose their value if they lose potency. In order to get the most out of your supplements, follow these simple guidelines:

* Store in a cool, dry place

* Keep the lid tightly sealed

* Pay attention to the expiration date

Time Release

These supplements release vitamins into your system gradually. While this sounds logical their value has been questioned. Ann Louise Gittelman, Ph.D., stated in the March 2000 issue of *Health Sciences Institute Members Alert*, that spacing out a number of vitamins several hours apart is just as effective if a steady flow throughout the day is your goal.

Supplements: Hold the Snake Oil Please

Everyone has heard the expression *caveat emptor*. Those words are Latin for *let the buyer beware.*

According to the PBS documentary *Frontline - The Alternative Fix*, nutritional supplements are currently an industry that rakes in over 15 billion dollars annually. Despite this fact, consumers don't always get what they pay for. The results of the studies listed below are food for thought:

An article published in the July 2001 issue of the *Journal of the American Medical Association* contained the results of a Vanderbilt University study of the popular herbal supplement St. John's Wort. The account of two hundred people suffering from depression showed the product to be an ineffective treatment for that condition.

A study done by *Consumer Reports* showed that brands of ginseng claiming to have the same concentration of the key ingredient actually varied widely, with some having up to ten times as much as others. In addition, some brands contained high levels of a wide variety of contaminants.

Some Promising Results

Below are several supplements that have shown great promise in fighting age related health concerns:

Coenzyme Q10: Also known as ubiquinone, Q10 has shown the ability to help keep aging arteries clear and to lower blood pressure. It aids in energy production and has demonstrated antioxidant properties. Q10 is also a booster of immune function.

Ginkgo Biloba: Has shown benefits in fighting Alzheimer's disease by increasing blood flow to the brain. Be mindful, however, of the serious side effects reported as the result of several studies. These include increased bleeding for those with clotting disorders and negative interactions with certain antidepressant medications.

Soy: The soybean contains compounds known as isoflavones, which once isolated, can be converted into the form of a supplement. Studies have shown these products to be effective in treating some symptoms suffered by menopausal women including hot flashes, mood swings and a reduction in cognitive function. There is also some evidence that soy supplements may protect against fractures and can lower levels of LDL. Be aware that these supplements have been rumored to increase the risk for breast cancer; however, those rumors have yet to be substantiated. To play it safe, limit soy supplementation in the form of isoflavones to no more than 160 mg per day.

Milk Thistle: Those suffering from liver ailments should take note of recent findings that have shown this herb to be an effective treatment for hepatitis B and C as well as cirrhosis.

Garlic: There is strong evidence that garlic protects us from heart disease by thinning the blood. This pungent herb also fights infections and detoxifies both the liver and colon. It may also help fight Alzheimer's disease. To avoid the strong flavor and smell of this powerful herb it is often converted into a supplement and consumed in pill form. Studies on garlic supplements have shown conflicting results and whether a garlic pill provides the same benefit as the herb itself remains a topic of debate.

Noni Juice: Made from the fruit of the Morinda citrifolia, a plant that is tropical in origin. Despite its strong aroma, noni juice is one of the most popular supplements on the market and has been hailed as a treatment for everything from a bad heart to bad breath. While the wild claims attributed to this product are hard to verify, its effectiveness in treating both pain and inflammation have been well documented.

Supplements to Avoid

The following section might be the most important part of this chapter. That is because taking one thing that's harmful can easily negate many positives. Below is a list of supplements whose potential benefits are far outweighed by their potential dangers. Also, be aware that some supplements that are safe for the general population may be a danger to people with certain health conditions or when combined with other supplements. Because of this, it is wise to consult either a doctor or qualified dietician before taking any supplement.

Androstenedione: Made famous by home run king Mark McGuire, andro, as it is known, is a steroid banned from most team sports. It is a precursor of testosterone that carries with it many of the same side effects as anabolic steroids. They include: shrinking of the testicles and impotence in men and increased risks of cancer, blood clots and the development of masculine characteristics in women. Teenagers also face an increased risk of both acne and stunted growth.

1,4-butanediol: Found in a number of different products aimed at everyone from bodybuilders to those looking to regrow their thinning hair, this supplement has been implicated in 71 deaths with still more under investigation. According to *The New England Journal of Medicine*, "...1,4-butanediol is toxic, addictive and potentially lethal."

Ephedra: First supplement to be banned by the FDA. Ephedra has been implicated in numerous deaths including former Oriole's pitcher Steve Bechler. It is sobering to note that at the time it was outlawed at least 62 companies were manufacturing ephedra products.

Bitter Orange: Contains synephrine, which is used in hospital emergency rooms to quickly raise the blood pressure of patients suffering from shock. Chemically, it is a close relative of ephedra, complete with many of the same dangers.

Others worth noting:

Kava and skullcap may cause liver damage and yohimbine can lead to changes in blood pressure, arrhythmia and respiratory depression.

Fat burners: Don't Get Burned!

"If something sounds too good to be true it usually is."

"There ain't no free lunch."

"You can't get something for nothing."

Each adage listed above shares the same age old wisdom, if you want results you'll have to work for them. This is particularly relevant today as countless consumers are seduced by the holy grail of all current supplements, the highly sought after "fat burner!" There are literally dozens of these concoctions sold everywhere you look, on TV, radio and in magazines and newspapers. They sound great. The pictures are quite impressive. The only problem is...They don't work! That's not to say you might not lose pounds and inches temporarily. Amphetamines have been offering you that option for years but at what cost? Of these products, the ones that work at all do so at the expense of lean muscle mass, the very substance that will allow you to lose weight properly.

Circumstances that Might Restrict Vitamin Intake

The following are several circumstances that may alter your nutritional requirements. If you have a specific health concern, then it is wise to check with your health care provider. They will be able to tailor your vitamin and mineral intake to your specific needs.

Pregnancy

Vitamin A is a powerful antioxidant but when taken in unusually high doses can lead to birth defects. Because of this, mega doses of vitamin A are contraindicated for those who are pregnant or may become pregnant.

Advanced Kidney Disease

People on dialysis quickly learn that they must not only restrict fluid intake, but intake of several essential minerals as well. These minerals include potassium, magnesium and phosphorous, or as one of my friends who suffers from this affliction philosophically put it, "All the things that other people need."

Men/Postmenopausal Women

Iron: Supplemental iron is important to premenopausal women. This is because menstruation robs them of much of their iron and that iron must be replaced. In order to maintain recommended levels of this important mineral, vitamins taken by women yet to reach menopause should contain approximately 10 milligrams of iron, 56 percent of the RDA. For the majority of men and postmenopausal women this is not the case. Too much iron can be damaging to your body, putting you at risk for heart or liver damage. This is due in part to iron's relationship with free radicals and their tendency to attack healthy cells. Because of this, men and postmenopausal women should take vitamins that are iron free, unless otherwise advised by their physician.

Those on Anticoagulant Medications

Certain individuals suffer from hypercoagulation, a tendency towards excess clotting of the blood. This condition can lead to stroke, heart attack or pulmonary embolus, life threatening conditions that are often treated with medication such as heparin or warfarin.

Some supplements that are also helpful in preventing these ailments should not be combined with anticoagulant medications. This is because they may cause the medication to work *too* well, leading to excessive bleeding and putting the individual at risk for a hemorrhagic stroke. These substances include vitamin E and fish oil and should not be taken by individuals who are taking anticoagulant medications without consulting their physician.

Aspirin

While aspirin is a drug and does not truly belong in the vitamin/ supplement section, since this book does not have a drug section I am including it here. Scientific study has proven that for many older people, particularly men, one baby aspirin taken daily can cut their heart attack risk by 50 percent. Because of this, over 40 million aspirins are taken by Americans each day for that purpose, a number roughly equal to the amount consumed for its original, painkilling function. Aspirin has also shown promise as a cancer fighting agent.

Despite its proven value, aspirin is still a drug, and when mixed with other drugs or supplements can sometimes result in a negative interaction. Examples include ginkgo biloba, as well as blood thinning medications such as coumadin. Always check with your physician before combining aspirin or any other drug with other medications.

Suggested Reading

Jean Carper's Total Nutrition Guide by Jean Carper (Bantam, March 1, 1987)

Nutrition Specialist Manual by Dr. Jane Pentz (LAM Pub, 4th ed edition, 1998)

Want More Info?

For those interested in more information on supplements, the American Nutraceutical Association has a website that could prove helpful. You can find it at: www.americanutra.com

Finally, for those serious about learning the latest ins and outs of this confusing topic, Dr. Pentz teaches a two day course that is quite informative and is offered in numerous cities throughout the country. Information is available on her website: www.lifestylemanagement.com.

"An ounce of prevention is worth a pound of cure."
—English Jurist Henry De Bracton

9 | 8:05 a.m.
Will You Use Sunscreen?

In the mid-eighties I became friendly with a bartender at a top New York night spot. The place hired only good-looking bartenders and my friend more than met the requirements. A few years passed, and after a long and successful career filled with every possible excess he decided to move to Florida for a change of pace. About a year later I went to visit him and was amazed by how much he had aged. In one year, the sun had done what twenty years on the New York club scene never could.

A few years later, I returned from a relaxing vacation at a beach locale. During my next visit to the gym the young lady behind the front desk heard where I'd been and asked, "Where's your tan?" I conveyed to her that getting skin cancer has never been one of my priorities, to which she again repeated, "Where's your tan?" At that point I just gave up. I've never forgotten that conversation. Partly because her inability to see my point of view amused me but also because it brought to the forefront how obsessed we are with tanning. To this woman, no other viewpoint was possible. She was about twenty at the time. I've often wondered how old she looks today.

Many people grew up thinking there was nothing better than darkening their skin through some fun in the sun. A tan was said to look *healthy*. Nothing could be further from the truth. The effects of the sun can be devastating. It ages us beyond our years and is a primary cause of skin cancer. Many people fail to realize that tanning is actually the result of damage done to your skin and its attempt to protect itself through the production of additional pigment.

The Psychology of Tanning

In order to better understand our tanning obsession, it's important to look at it from a historical perspective. In Victorian times, darkened skin was actually frowned upon. It was viewed as a sign that one was a working stiff since most manual labor was done outdoors. Those who were wealthy could merely sit around under a parasol, sipping tea and chatting about those less fortunate. Then modern technology changed all that. As machinery started taking over many tasks once performed by hand, a high percentage of jobs shifted indoors. Now, those with means were on the beach vacationing while the poor working stiffs toiled in the cold, cruel mailroom or in front of their computer. The reality of our desire to darken has little to do with it looking better and a lot to do with giving the impression of wealth. *That* is the basis of our tanning obsession.

Location, Location, Location

As my fair skinned friend found out, Miami is not New York. The closer you get to the equator the more harmful the sun's UV rays become. They also bounce off both sand and water making continuous fun in the sun a risky choice. But the beach is not the only culprit. High altitude increases the danger as does wind and snow, so skiing in Aspen is just as good a reason to protect yourself.

Conditions Resulting from Too Much Sun

Sun Poisoning: Prolonged exposure to the sun during the time when ultraviolet rays are at their highest concentration can lead to this painful condition typified by a red rash and/or blistering of the skin. It is especially common among diabetics, those suffering from infections or those who have had it previously. Certain drugs which increase ones sensitivity to ultraviolet light can also be a factor.

Heat Cramps: Caused by exercising in a hot, humid environment. This condition often leads to muscle spasms.

Heat Exhaustion: This is another common condition that affects those exercising in a hot, humid environment. Its symptoms include profuse sweating, depressed blood pressure, loss of coordination, nausea and vomiting.

Heat Stroke: Also known as sunstroke, this condition, resulting from prolonged exposure to high temperatures, is considered a medical emergency. Symptoms include hot dry skin, rapid pulse and elevated body temperature; left unchecked may result in brain damage, coma or death. If you suspect that you or someone you know may be suffering from heat stroke, medical treatment should be sought immediately.

Tanning Salons: A Safer Alternative?

The answer to this question is a resounding no! In fact, research has shown tanning beds to be far *more* dangerous than the sun itself. According to a study conducted at New York's Mount Sinai School of Medicine, tanning beds subject the body to levels of cancer causing ultraviolet rays that are between ten and fifteen times higher than those given off by the sun. To make matters worse, most tanning salons use ultraviolet-A bulbs to darken the skin of their clientele. While ultraviolet-B rays can be harmful, it is the UVA rays that are more dangerous, due to their deeper penetration of the skin.

What to Do?

Nothing will stop all the sun's effects but there are protective measures that can be taken to minimize the damage. A primary line of defense is the regular use of sunscreen. "Sunscreen helps prevent all those things that people worry about when they grow older, i.e., wrinkles, brown spots and loose skin," says Dr. Steven Simon, a New York dermatologist, "Its good preventive medicine." Assuming you agree that your skin is worth saving, then choosing the right product is equally important.

SPF

We've all seen the letters SPF on bottles of sunscreen yet many people don't fully understand what they mean. SPF stands for sun protection factor, a number that tells you how long you can be exposed to the sun before being burned. An SPF of 15 means that you could spend approximately 15 times as long in the sun before burning as you could if unprotected. For those who can handle 15 minutes of exposure before changing color, an SPF of 15 should extend that grace period to a little over three and one half hours, at which point it must be reapplied. Keep in mind that both swimming and excessive perspiration reduce the time period during which the sunscreen you've applied will remain effective. Because of this, more frequent application is a good idea. Since your sunscreen's SPF number only applies to its level of protection against the sun's UVB rays make sure the product you choose has UVA protection as well. Also be aware that while sunscreens with an SPF of 50 or more are available, their level of protection can be misleading. Since all sunscreens allow some of the sun's rays to penetrate, no product provides total protection. If you want to look young don't press your luck!

Choosing Between Every Brand Under the Sun

In a world filled with hype, choosing the right brand can be a challenge. There are dozens of formulas on the market, each being touted as the newest or best. Below are a couple of products you might want to consider. While they are by no means the only good choices available, they are recommended by many dermatologists.

For your face you might try NeoStrata. It combines sunscreen with a moisturizer to provide additional benefit. On your arms and other exposed areas, Ti-Silc is a good choice. It features sun block 45 but unlike NeoStrata does not contain a moisturizer. While an SPF of 45 may seem high, make sure that the brand you choose has a number of 15 or above. It should also include one of several ingredients that have been proven effective: titanium dioxide, zinc oxide or avobenzone. If your sunscreen has one of these compounds it is more likely to be a quality product.

If you are looking for an even higher SPF, another favorite of many dermatologists is Neutrogena Ultra Sheer Dry-Touch Sunblock SPF 55. It is effective yet lacks the greasiness of other products with equally high SPFs.

Remember, whichever brand you choose, apply the product liberally. Studies have shown that most people use far less sunscreen than is recommended.

How Long Has This Been Going On?

How old is your current bottle of suntan lotion? If you use this product year round (as you should), and if it has lasted more than two months, you are probably not using enough. If you choose to use it only during the summer months or when on vacation, a large bottle can last considerably longer. Sunscreen more than a year old is probably past its prime. Expiration dates are printed on these products and should be checked before coating yourself with a false sense of security.

Other Safety Measures

Hats and sunglasses are recommended, as are umbrellas, particularly when on the beach, where both water and sand magnify the sun's damaging rays. Another common-sense solution, particularly in places where the sun is quite strong, is to avoid exposure during the hours when the sun is at its most intense, generally between 10 a.m. and 4 p.m.

Self-tanning Lotions: The Way to Go?

Self-tanning lotions work by interacting with proteins in your skin. Unlike the sun or a tanning bed, self-tanners provide the results you're seeking without the risk of cancer or a damaged immune system. While these products once gave users an extremely artificial looking tan, the technology has improved and is now a viable option.

Suggested Reading

Don't Go to the Cosmetics Counter Without Me by Paula Begoun (Beginning Press, 6th edition January 2003)

It's Not Just About Wrinkles: A Park Avenue Dermatologist's Program for Beautiful Skin—in Just Four Minutes a Day by Neal B. Schultz MD (Stewart, Tabori and Chang, June 1, 2006)

The Wrinkle Cure by Nicholas Perricone (Warner Books, 2001)

Want More Info?

The American Academy of Dermatology is a good choice. Visit their website at: www.aad.org.

Paula Begoun hosts a site that contains great info on sunscreen as well as many other aspects of skincare. You can find it at: www.cosmeticscop.com.

The Sun and Your Eyes

Using sunscreen is a great way to limit damage to your skin, but what about your eyes? Exposure to sunlight is a factor in the development of macular degeneration, the leading cause of vision loss for Americans fifty and older. It also plays a role in the development of cataracts. Below are a few steps you can take to insure that you will be able to see that skin you're working so hard to protect:

*Limit exposure: Here more is *definitely* not better. Try to minimize your time of exposure, especially during peak hours or in tropical climates.

*Sunglasses: Not all eye wear is created equal. Wear 100 percent ultraviolet blocking sunglasses.

*Hats: Wearing a hat, especially one with a wide brim, offers your eyes added protection.

*Don't Smoke: When it comes to macular degeneration, smoking is also a contributing factor. It impairs circulation, thereby decreasing the supply of blood to the retina. Smoking also makes you three times as likely to develop cataracts. So while you're out there in all that fresh air and sunshine, why not find a trash can in which to deposit the remainder of your supply?

"Music washes away from the soul the dust of everyday life."
—Red Auerbach

"Music is the wine that fills the cup of silence."
—Robert Fripp

10 8:10 a.m. Will You Start Your Day With Music?

In 1986, I dated a woman who made a point of listening to one of her favorite songs everyday, just before leaving the house. We didn't date for long, but that concept, a simple logical idea, stuck with me. According to a Penn State study, whatever type of music you choose to listen to will improve your mood. In another study done in Michigan and Florida involving 130 retirees, most claimed that taking keyboard lessons greatly diminished feelings of anxiety, depression and loneliness. Improving your mood reduces stress and thereby reduces illness. That's being proactive.

Music is being used by an ever increasing number of hospitals to help patients cope with the trauma of surgery. In November 2000, a musician named Kate Richards dealt with her childhood fear of surgery by listening to music immediately before and after the operation. She described her recovery room experience as follows, "I somehow felt my nerves were being massaged."

Pablo Casals

"I despise a world which does not feel that music is a higher revelation than all wisdom and philosophy."
—Ludwig van Beethoven

To see how music can improve your quality of life you need look no further than legendary cellist, Pablo Casals. In the mid-1960s author Norman Cousins visited Casals at his home in Puerto Rico. He noted how the maestro, then almost 90 years of age, appeared as he first arose, with his posture badly stooped, his fingers swollen and clinched, and his breathing labored. Don Pablo always started his day at the piano, playing classics penned by Bach and Brahms. Cousins watched in amazement as beautiful music flowed from fingers that seemed incapable of tying a shoe just moments before. Soon all the aforementioned maladies miraculously improved, allowing the elderly man to move freely and with ease. Cousins detailed the experience in his best selling book, *Anatomy of an Illness as Perceived by the Patient.*

Music Therapy

Music therapy is a discipline that uses music in a clinical setting to treat a wide variety of conditions. The American Music Therapy Association (AMTA) defines it as, "The clinical and evidence-based use of music interventions to accomplish individualized goals within a therapeutic relationship by a credentialed professional who has completed an approved music therapy program."

Today many hospitals, nursing homes and rehabilitation clinics employ music therapists to improve the physical and mental health of their patients. Some of the conditions it is used to treat include:

Alzheimer's disease: Music therapy has been used to treat Alzheimer's patients and has been effective in improving their ability to function both physically and mentally. According to Al Bumanis, MT-BC, AMTA Director of Communications, "Music therapy gives the Alzheimer's patient a sense of reality by bringing back parts of the personality that are gone most of the time."

Parkinson's disease: Parkinson's is a condition that affects over a million and one half Americans. Symptoms include tremors, difficulty walking and movements that are slow or rigid. Music Therapy has shown great promise in treating Parkinson's patients. The ability to feel and react to rhythm has enabled sufferers to initiate movements that would have otherwise proved difficult or impossible.

Stress and Pain Management: When listing strategies to cope with the damaging effects of both stress and pain, music is often included. By listening and breathing to music, sufferers are often able to reduce their medication. In a hospital setting music is especially useful. According to Mr. Bumanis, "If you relax the patient, then certain procedures are easier to do."

Depression: Music is especially useful in treating depression, since those afflicted find this method of treatment non-threatening. According to Mr. Bumanis, "It is a way to communicate with clients when other things don't work."

Qualifications

In order to qualify as a music therapist, a college degree in the field is required. A candidate must also pass the national examination offered by the Certification Board for Music Therapists. Once those requirements have been met the individual is considered a board certified music therapist or MT-BC.

Want More Info?

Visit the American Music Therapy Association website located at: www.musictherapy.org.

New Age Music: Hype or Healing?

I've often attended the New Life Expo, a holistic health fair held twice a year. On those occasions, sandwiched between a collection of massage therapists and aromatherapy proponents, was someone selling music said to heal. Whether these claims are exaggerated or not is hard to either prove or disprove. Still, it is safe to say, that New Age music relieves stress and promotes an overall feeling of well being.

Choosing a Title

Musical taste varies widely and in that respect the New Age variety is no different. Some enjoy gentle acoustic guitar rhythms or airy sounds flowing from an electronic keyboard. Others prefer stronger, more tribal rhythms or sounds from nature that hardly resemble traditional music at all. Whichever the case, for music to be considered New Age, it should share a common thread, to lift the spirit and rejuvenate the mind and body.

Below are some of my personal favorites. They may not be your taste, but if you are not familiar with the genre, they will give you a place to start.

Majesty by Aeoliah: One of my earliest purchases of New Age music. I first heard it playing in a store in Greenwich Village accompanied by a video of scenes from nature. They went so well together that I thought they came that way. I bought this so long ago that I have it on cassette. Wonder if anyone has the 8-track lying around somewhere?

Angel Love by Aeoliah: The back of the CD states that, *"Angel Love* was conceived primarily as a musical offering to help us attune to the healing energies and harmonious emotions of the angelic kingdom." Now if that's not New Age I don't know what is! Whatever you call it, I find its forty five minutes of soothing sounds to be far too short.

Midnight Flower by Drala: I find this jazzy creation to be quite hypnotic and since it has more of a beat than some of the more ethereal New Age selections, it might not sound as strange to the neighbors. For trivia buffs: David Nichtern, a member of Drala, is also the author of Maria Muldaur's seventies hit *Midnight at The Oasis.*

Simple Massage by Brian Tay: Originally released as *Garden Rain*, this CD comes with a set of cards offering massage tips. This combination of rainfall and light music is as relaxing as anything I have ever heard. I play it on those occasions when I have trouble falling asleep and have never been awake to hear it end.

Inner Peace by Steven Halpern: You can't get more relaxing than this. Has a light tone, even for this type of music. Halpern is also the author of, *Sound Health: The Music and Sounds That Make Us Whole.*

How Music Heals

The fact that music improves our health by bringing us pleasure, and relieving stress is undeniable. But does it heal in other, more tangible ways? Much has been written in the holistic health community about the therapeutic value of the types of music listed below. Whether their benefits are exaggerated is hard to say, but at minimum they merit further study.

Chanting

Chanting can be defined as the repetition of a monotonous musical phrase, often with a religious or otherwise spiritual connotation. Done for centuries in numerous cultures throughout the world, chanting is believed by many to heal the body and elevate the spirit. Below are several types of chanting that have been used for therapeutic purposes:

Gregorian Chants: Attributed to monks of Medieval Europe, these unaccompanied melodies, sung in Latin, are named after Pope Gregory I. In his book *Healing Sounds*, Jonathan Goldman relates how the monks of a Benedictine monastery were for a time forbidden to chant.

The monks grew ill and did not regain their health until they resumed their practice of chanting six to eight hours per day.

Throat Singing: In Tuva, an area that borders Mongolia, a type of music called hoomi, or throat singing, is an integral part of the culture. Here, two notes, one high and flutelike, the other much deeper in pitch, are sung by the same person simultaneously. Throat singing makes substantial use of harmonics and is believed by many to have great therapeutic value.

One Voice Chords: Developed in fifteenth century Tibet by the monks of the Gyume Tantric monastery and Gyoto Tantric College, this style of music remained a mystery to the outside world for hundreds of years. It enables an individual to form chords by singing three notes simultaneously. Unlike throat singing, which makes use of wordless melodies, the Tibetan monks work sacred text into the chants that they create.

Harmonics

Whenever you hit a musical note, other related tones are also brought into play. These "overtones" are located at specific intervals in relation to the original note or "fundamental" and are also called harmonics. Many, who believe strongly in the healing power of sound, have a great interest in the potential benefits that harmonics have to offer.

Entrainment

The law of vibration states that all things vibrate at all times. This is true of the blades of grass growing beneath your feet, the lawn chair you've placed on them, and you yourself as you sit there enjoying a warm summer day. Many believe that when a part of your body is ill, it no longer vibrates at the proper resonance. By exposing yourself to strong vibrations from an object that is at the correct frequency, some believe that the weaker object's vibrations can become synchronized with those of the stronger. This is the concept of entrainment.

Singing Bowls

An example of the therapeutic use of both harmonics and entrainment can be heard and felt in the form of the Tibetan singing bowls. These metal bells, shaped like bowls, have been used for centuries throughout Asia to heal and assist in the practice of meditation. By striking the bowl with a wooden mallet both sound and vibrations are produced that many believe have healing properties. The mallet can also be run around the rim of the bowl to increase the sound's duration. Bowls are usually made of metal, often bronze, but those made of crystal are also available. Debate rages on as to which instrument provides the greatest benefit.

Pump *Down* the Volume?

Playing in rock bands was a great experience, but everything has its price. About ten years ago I noticed that I wasn't hearing as well as I once had. A hearing test revealed that I had suffered a hearing loss in a certain high frequency band. While music can help to keep you young, who wants to be young and deaf?

Ear Plugs: The Song Remains the Same, Just Quieter

From train conductors and construction workers, to the drummer in a thrash metal band, this invention can help save both your hearing and your sanity. There are many different models to choose from. They range from two pieces of foam that pop out of a vending machine and cost about a dollar, to the Cadillac of ear plugs which are purchased from a medical professional and custom fitted to your ear. The expensive ones don't block out everything but instead limit only the sounds that are damaging. The downside is that they cost about two hundred dollars and need to be replaced periodically.

Suggested Reading

Healing Sounds: The Power of Harmonics by Jonathan Goldman (Healing Arts Press, 3rd edition, June 30, 2002)

The Healing Power of Sound: Recovery from Life-Threatening Illness Using Sound, Voice, and Music by Mitchell L. Gaynor, M.D. (Shambhala, Reprint edition, August 13, 2002)

The New Music Therapist's Handbook by Suzanne B. Hanser (Berklee Press Publications, 2nd edition, March 1, 2000)

Want More Info?

The Sound Healers Association (SHA) is an organization dedicated to the use of sound and music for therapeutic purposes. You can visit their website at: www.soundhealersassociation.org.

"A dog is man's best friend."
—Unknown

"One touch of nature makes the whole world kin."
—From *Troilus and Cressida* by William Shakespeare

11 | 8:15 a.m.
Will You Pet the Dog?

I recall waiting in line to enter a trendy night club, fronted by an obnoxious doorman. As anyone who has had that experience can tell you, it can be a bit annoying. Just as I began feeling somewhat stressed, a woman came walking by with her pet greyhound. She needed to go into a store for a moment and asked if I'd mind watching Casey. It took her about five minutes during which time I petted the pup to take his mind off the temporary loss of his owner. When she returned I noticed something quite remarkable, the stress I had been feeling was gone. She thanked me for watching him, but in reality I should have thanked her, or more appropriately, Casey.

In the winter of 2006, I went for a series of ten Rolfing sessions. Rolfing is a type of deep tissue bodywork that can be quite painful at times. During one especially grueling session the Rolfer's cat decided to jump up on the massage table and lie down next to me. I soon began to pet her with my free hand and before long became less aware of the pain, a plus when someone has their elbow dug, what feels like two inches, into your spine.

Having a Pet

"Whoever said you can't buy happiness forgot about puppies."
—Gene Hill

Numerous studies have shown that pets reduce stress levels, which leads to a longer, healthier life. Here are some interesting findings:

Pets and Blood Pressure: In a University of Pennsylvania study, researchers found that watching fish swim in a home aquarium can be an effective way to treat high blood pressure.

In another conducted by Dr. Karen Allen of the State University of New York at Buffalo, she studied the effects of owning a pet, on members of one of the most stressful professions of all, stockbroker. Those involved were taking drugs to control their blood pressure and by the end of the study almost 50 percent of them were able to discard their medication.

Pets and Depression: Exposure to animals can instantly change the mood of those who are clinically depressed, eliciting a response from individuals who often remain unresponsive. More on the use of animals in treating depression will be listed in the pet therapy section of this chapter.

Pets and Heart Disease: In a study performed by Dr. Allen, she discovered that owning a pet improved the survival rate of heart attack victims. In another conducted at a New York City hospital, patient's progress was followed after their release. It was found that the survival rate of pet owning patients was significantly higher than it was for those who did not have one. Keep that in mind as you head for work, and remember to pet the dog. As for the fish... maybe just wave.

How Does It Work?

The Joys of Heavy Petting: In an article written by Marty Becker, DVM, he discusses the physiological effect of petting. He reports that when a person pets a dog or cat a slew of beneficial hormones are released into their system. As a result of this their levels of cortisol, a stress hormone, are reduced. He described the results as, "A biochemical spa treatment of sorts."

Unconditional Love: One of finest attributes that a dog possesses is consistency. It doesn't matter if Fido had a bad hair day or if you forgot his birthday, the pup jumps out of his skin to greet you the moment you enter the room. Knowing that a friend who loves you is waiting at home makes that rush hour commute much more bearable.

Dogs and Cancer

> *"A dog has the soul of a philosopher."*
> **—Plato**

When you talk about the enemies of a long and healthy life, cancer is at the top of the list. It is a disease that effects people of all ages but the older we get the worse our odds seem to be. Not only does the disease itself ravage our bodies, but so does the cure. The earlier it is caught the better the odds of survival and the less debilitating the treatment. That leads to the question, can dogs diagnose cancer? Until recently that claim would have been viewed as bizarre to say the least, however, several well publicized studies have pointed to the possible use of dog's acute sense of smell as a tool in the early diagnosis of breast, lung and bladder cancer. In one study, five dogs were trained to detect breast cancer and were 88 percent successful. When it came to lung cancer the results were better still. Studies conducted in Great Britain also found that dogs were successful in the diagnosis of bladder cancer. While it's too early to throw away your doctor's business card and head for the nearest kennel, these studies are hard to ignore, and point once again to the ways in which animals enrich our lives.

Can't Own a Pet?

Some people are not in a position to take in a furry or feathered companion; your building won't allow it, your apartment is too small, your wife has allergies or your life is just too hectic to care for one properly. Don't fret; there are still many ways to work the joy and benefit of pets into your daily life.

Pet Therapy

> *"Animals are such agreeable friends - they ask*
> *no questions, they pass no criticisms."*
> **—George Eliot**

In order to fully appreciate the therapeutic value of animals all you need do is read about pet therapy, which uses exposure to animals to treat a wide variety of ailments. "Pet Therapy can be effective in treating just about any illness," according to Michelle Cobey of the Delta Society, an organization that registers both animals and handlers. Animals from guinea pigs to llamas have been registered with the society and are brought into hospitals or nursing homes to raise the spirits of the sick and the elderly.

The effectiveness of therapy animals, especially dogs, in treating depression is quite remarkable. People often become more alert and active in their presence. The simple act of petting, taken for granted by most of us, has added value for those who are bedridden. Immobility often becomes a vicious cycle, leading to further debilitation. The small increase in movement that petting provides not only improves their mood but also speeds their recovery.

The requirements to become either a therapy animal or its handler are not mandated by law; they are set by various certifying bodies such as the Delta Society. Upon meeting the requirements, the Delta Society has a two year fee of seventy five dollars which not only registers both the handler and animal, but also provides the handler with liability insurance. Each facility making use of this service decides which certifications they are willing to accept.

If you're interested in getting more information on pet therapy, the Delta Society has a fine website. It offers scientifically based articles touting the benefits of pet therapy as well as plenty of information on how to get involved, either as a volunteer or as the recipient of such services. Visit them at: www.deltasociety.org. Another great resource is Dog Play. Its website has a page with dozens of links that are full of relevant information. Visit them at: www.dogplay.com.

Other People's Pets

I'm that guy you see walking down the street who stops to play with other people's dogs. I tend to be cautious, not wanting to impose myself on others, but more times than not the proud owner ends up beaming and I'm happy having spent a moment with my new furry friend. Usually the dog seems happy too, so everybody wins!

It appears that I'm not alone. On January 2, 2006, the *New York Post* ran a story about a dog named Jake, a terrier who spends much of his time backstage at New York's famed Lincoln Center. For ten years, he's received kudos from some of the world's most accomplished musicians for calming their nerves as well as cheering up those who've had a bad night.

A word of caution: Remember to always ask, (the owner not the dog), before playing with an animal that you are not familiar with. In addition to being polite, this could save you from a painful bite. Being bitten by an animal will definitely not lengthen your life and in the case of a sick one, might shorten it considerably.

The Zoo

When caring for a pet on a daily basis isn't practical, a trip to your local zoo can be a wonderful substitute. A far cry from the cruel animal prisons of days gone by, the modern zoo is as comfortable for its residents as it is enjoyable for those of us on the other side of the glass. Consider joining your local zoological society. Many offer substantial benefits including members-only nights, discounts on educational programs and a newsletter. You may also develop a colorful collection of tee shirts, often a bonus when rejoining. To find a location near you, visit Sarah's Zoo Page at: www.mindspring.com/~brucec/zoo.htm.

The Petting Zoo

If you like getting close to our animal friends, then consider a trip to your local petting zoo. Once there, you can feed and fawn over a variety of species ranging from fairly common, to quite exotic. At the Smoky Mountain Deer Farm & Exotic Petting Zoo, located in Sevierville, Tennessee, you can feed and pet a zebra. Paws and Claws in Hawley, Pennsylvania, has a camel that loves making new friends and a giraffe that eats right out of your hand. SeaWorld in San Diego, California, has a petting pool for dolphins. For an international listing of petting zoos, visit the following website: www.pettingzoofarm.com.

Animal Planet

Launched in 1996, Animal Planet is a network filled with shows that both amuse and inform. Featured programs include, *Crocodile Hunter*, starring the late Steve Erwin, *Meerkat Manor* and *The Planet's Funniest Animals*. For a full program guide, visit their website at: www.animal. discovery.com.

Animal Pageants

On May 14, 2006, the second annual *Bulldog Beauty Contest* was held in Long Beach, California. Over 100 entrants were judged by several two-legged beauty pageant winners, on their confidence and character, as well as that unmistakable bulldog smile. Whether it's Cincinnati's *Ferret Buckeye Bash* or *Halloween with Horses* held annually in Parker, Colorado, animal pageants can be just the ticket for critter lovers without a pet of their own. A wide variety of contests are held nationwide for everything from pugs to hermit crabs. Keep your eyes open for an event near you.

Suggested Reading

The Simon and Schuster Encyclopedia of Animals by Philip Whitfield (Simon & Schuster, November 2, 1998)

The Healing Power of Pets: Harnessing the Ability of Pets to Make and Keep People Happy and Healthy by Marty Becker (Hyperion, 1st edition, February 6, 2002)

Suggested Viewing

Animals Are Beautiful People (1974)
Babe (1995)
The Bear (1985)
March of the Penguins (2005)
Milo and Otis (1986)

"A place for everything and everything in its place"
—Benjamin Franklin

12 | 8:20 a.m.
Are You Stifled By Clutter?

In 1998, I finally convinced my 79 year-old father to sell the house he could no longer care for and move to Florida. Before he could do so, I had to go about a task I would wish on no man or beast; that of cleaning out his backyard and garage. My father had a scary tendency to keep everything and I mean *everything*. While working my way through the garage I found the detachable hood of an old winter coat. I was about to toss it in the trash pile when much to my surprise he informed me that he might still need it. It had no coat to attach it to and he was moving to South Florida where the temperature rarely dips below 70. When I asked him why, he said it was good when it snowed—*in Miami*? Another of his prized possessions was a barbecue he'd built in the backyard 40 years earlier. He loved to tell everyone how he barbequed with natural wood. The only problem was you couldn't get near the barbeque because the wood was in the way. This wasn't *really* a problem since he hadn't used it in over 30 years.

In retrospect, these stories about my Dad can be amusing. Unfortunately, they also represent a mindset that led to the depression and associated downward spiral that eventually ended his life.

That being said, I have a confession; I'm a packrat. As a writer I need a lot of reference material but I keep *way* more than I need. It may seem harmless, but in reality, clutter can be stifling. It bogs us down both physically and mentally and the more it piles up the harder it is to deal with. Webster's New World Dictionary defines clutter as, "A number of things scattered in disorder, jumble." When put in those terms a pile of papers sitting on my table doesn't sound all that appealing. Let's look at what it has in store for us.

The Physical

Dust and Mold

One of the problems with unnecessary clutter is the dust that it collects. Dust contains many substances including pollen and animal dander, to which many people are allergic. Dust is not only irritating but can cause asthma, a potentially serious health condition.

Some types of clutter, paper in particular, can cause mold to form as it decays. Mold can further impair your health by damaging your respiratory system. This is a major concern since stacks of paper are one of the most common forms of clutter. So on your way out the door today, gather up those old newspapers, toss out that Woodstock tee shirt that's now three sizes too small and make some floor or counter space to accommodate the cage for the new ferret you've been longing for since finishing chapter eleven.

All Creatures, Small and Smaller Still

When I recommended pets this was *not* what I meant. One problem with clutter, particularly paper or cardboard, is the "crowd" that it attracts. All manner of creepies and crawlies tend to set up shop turning a harmless pile of papers into their personal condo. Insects and rodents find paper, especially damp paper, quite inviting. Furthermore, hungry mice have no reservations about turning it into a between-meal snack.

FIRE!

While the last several paragraphs covered some aspects of clutter that can be annoying or even unhealthy, they don't compare to this possible consequence. While mice like paper wet, fire prefers it dry as kindling and can quickly turn a pile of apparently harmless clutter, as well as your home, into an inferno. Be especially careful around radiators, stoves and candles along with any other source of high heat or open flame.

The Emotional

The reality is that the emotional toll taken by clutter far outweighs the physical. Having junk all around you is stifling and tends to cause a vicious cycle of lethargy which leads to more clutter in much the way inactivity leads to more inactivity. Breaking the cycle will help you take back possession of both your home and life and will prove to be a truly liberating experience. Give it a try!

Tips for Avoiding or Eliminating Clutter

*Go Through Your Mail Immediately: Many busy people bring all of their mail upstairs, toss it on the table and figure they'll get around to it eventually. Big Mistake.

*Give Away Clothes: Why stuff your closet with clothing that no longer fits or you will never wear again? There are people who can benefit from items that are no longer of use to you. This will also make room in your closet for the garments that you purchased after reading chapter four.

*Donate Old Books and Magazines: Save those that you use for reference, or that have strong sentimental value. Still, many people hang on to books that they haven't thought of in years and will never read again. Donating them to a library can do a good turn for others as well as bring you a tidy tax write-off. Another option is selling them to a used book store for a more immediate source of cash.

*Hire a Professional Organizer: These folks can help the more disorganized among us to get our act in gear. There is even a group dedicated to helping you find the one who is right for you. They are called the National Association of Professional Organizers (NAPO). You can visit their website at: www.napo.net.

*Have a Garage or Yard Sale: There is nothing like getting a few bucks for sitting in front of your house on a nice sunny day while ridding yourself of items you no longer want or need. Getting to know your neighbors better is an added plus.

Suggested Reading

One Thing at a Time: 100 simple ways to live Clutter-Free Every Day by Cindy Glovinsky, M.S.W., A.C.S.W. (St. Martin's Griffin, July 1, 2004)

Lighten Up!: Free Yourself from Clutter by Michelle Passoff (Harper Paperbacks, March 11, 1998)

Clear Your Desk! by Declan Treacy (Random House Business Books, April 1991)

Want More Info?

The following websites may be helpful to those wishing to clean up their act:

Messies Anonymous: www.messies.com.

Clutterers Anonymous (CLA): www.clutterersanonymous.net.

Feng Shui

Feng Shui is neither a method of hand-to-hand combat nor a type of sushi. It is an art originated in China, that can help us deal with our clutter. In her book, *Clear Your Clutter with Feng Shui*, Karen Kingston defines it as, "The art of balancing and harmonizing the flow of natural energies in our surroundings to create beneficial effects in our lives." As I glance at the stack of newspapers lounging on my kitchen table or the clothes on my dresser, which are choosing sides before making a run for the laundry bag, this sounds like just what the doctor ordered.

While many concepts are covered in the art of Feng Shui, such as proper furniture placement and the avoidance of downward hanging items in the homes of those who are prone to depression, for the purpose of expediency we will limit our focus to its principles in regard to clutter. According to Feng Shui practitioner Kathy Browning, "Clutter is trapped energy that has a far-reaching effect physically, mentally, emotionally and spiritually. Clutter makes you feel unorganized, confused, keeps you in the past, congests the body and leaves you feeling lethargic and tired. Clutter is energy constipation and who needs that?"

In her writing, Ms. Browning offers many useful tips on clearing clutter based on Feng Shui philosophy. One example is making a list of all the unfinished things in your life, claiming that allowing them to remain unfinished drains your energy. She also suggests donating books you no longer use, since they represent who you were in the past.

Those who practice Feng Shui believe that each part of your home represents an aspect of your life. While one area might correspond to your finances, another might represent your health or your reputation. It is believed that clutter in a given area negatively impacts the part of your existence that is aligned with it. Because of this, they feel that getting rid of items that are broken or that you no longer have use for will improve one or more aspects of your life.

A word of caution: as you work diligently to free your life of clutter, don't fill your home with piles of books on the subject. If you do choose to read up on Feng Shui, below are a few good choices:

Clear Your Clutter With Feng Shui by Karen Kingston (Broadway Books, 1998)

Feng Shui for Abundant Living by Kathy Browning (Kathy Browning, 2005)

Feng Shui For Dummies by David Daniel Kennedy (John Wiley & Sons Inc., 2000)

The Western Guide to Feng Shui: Creating Balance, Harmony, and Prosperity in Your Environment by Terah Kathryn Collins (Hay House, March 1996)

The Internet

If you'd like to keep in the Feng Shui spirit, information and the latest research is available on the following websites:

Feng Shui Research Center - www.astro-fengshui.com

SpiritualMinds.com - www.spiritualminds.com/fengshui.asp

Life Design Strategies - www.lifedesignstrategies.com/Articles.html

"A journey of a thousand miles begins with a single step."
—Lao-tzu, Chinese Philosopher

13 8:25 a.m. Will You Take The Stairs?

I live on the fifth floor of a seven-story building and routinely take the stairs. One day upon entering the lobby, I was greeted by a sign informing us that the elevator was out of order. Standing nearby a woman was cursing up a storm at the inconvenience to which she was being subjected. I have rarely seen anyone so upset. I was amazed to learn that she only lived on the second floor.

For people who get little or no exercise, regularly skipping an elevator ride in favor of a few flights of stairs can add years to your life. Still many people seem to have a strong aversion to it.

Benefits

* Runners will find that stair climbing offers similar cardiovascular benefit while at the same time reducing impact to the knees

* Since it is a weight-bearing activity, stair climbing fights osteoporosis by helping to build and maintain bone mass

* Stair climbing is a great way to prepare yourself for an emergency situation where your elevator is unavailable

Excuses

Everyone who avoids taking the stairs has a reason. Below are two popular ones along with why they don't hold water:

- **The Elevator Saves Time:** If your apartment is right next to the elevator and it's sitting there waiting for you maybe. If not, and you live no higher than the sixth or seventh floor, then the time you save will be minimal. It may even take you longer. I have often hit the stairs as one of my neighbors began waiting for the elevator. More often than not, we reached the lobby at the same time.

- **You're Too Tired:** Maybe, but do you want to stay that way? Lethargy is a vicious cycle leading you down a road to more unhealthy inactivity. I've even seen people take the elevator in the gym! It's easy to do nothing but what's easy is not always what's best. You're two flights up, come on, Push Yourself!

Take it to the Limit?

For those who seek the benefits of stair climbing in a competitive atmosphere, there are numerous stair climbing races held annually in over 80 locations around the world. One of the best known is New York's Empire State Building Run-up. This grueling event covers 1,576 steps that encompass 86 floors. For those interested in stair racing, the following website is a great resource:
www.towerrunning.com/english/races.htm.
It lists details of a variety of stair races held around the world.

Stair-Climbing Tips

*Maintain an Upright Posture:** Many people have a tendency to hunch their backs and lean forward when either climbing or descending a flight of stairs. This is bad for your back and should be avoided.

*Be Aware of Your Surroundings:** Stair climbing is great for your health but not if you slip on a wet spot or trip over a pile of garbage. Also be aware that not all steps are solid or all handrails firmly attached. A special note to women: staircases can sometimes become a second home to the criminal element. Be cautious of who may be lurking on the stairs you choose to climb.

*Watch Your Knees:** If you have a history of knee problems make sure to check with your doctor before adding stair climbing into your daily routine.

*Don't Overdo It:** As with other forms of exercise, it pays to start slowly. For a healthy person walking down from the third floor, this should not be an issue. On the other hand, a sedentary individual who has decided to start their stair climbing program by walking up 50 flights should consider a more conservative approach. A general guideline is to increase your distance about 10 percent per week.

Suggested Reading

The Relationship of Self-efficacy and Perceived Well-being to Physical Activity and Stair Climbing in Older Adults. : An article from: Research Quarterly for Exercise and Sport [HTML] by Diane L. Gill, Betty C. Kelley, Kathleen Williams and Jeffrey J. Martin (Amazon.com)

"Life is in the breath; therefore he who only half breathes, half lives."
—A Yogic proverb

"As I breathe deeply, I feel myself thrive. Thriving is as natural as breathing itself. By relaxing often, and breathing deeply your natural thriving is enhanced."
—Abraham

14 | 8:30 a.m. How Will You Breathe?

You've just finished climbing down the stairs and you're breathing pretty heavily. Breathing is something that's taken for granted by most everyone but how you breathe is a key factor in how well, and long, you live. The air around you provides oxygen, a substance that you cannot live without. If you deprive your brain of oxygen, its cells will begin to die within five minutes. In his book, *The 100 Simple Secrets of Healthy People*, author David Niven, PH.D., states, "Proper breathing is probably the easiest and most powerful way to protect your health. It results in better digestion and circulation, more restful sleep, decreased anxiety, and a more stable heart rate." So during your trip to work take a few minutes and focus on your breathing.

Problems

Are You Breathing in Reverse?

While that may seem like an odd question, the way many people breathe is actually backwards. When you inhale your rib cage should expand as your diaphragm descends. As you exhale your ribs should move down and in as your diaphragm rises. Surprisingly many people do the opposite. This is known as paradoxical breathing. There are few bodily processes we would do in reverse and still expect to fully benefit. Think of your lungs as if they were balloons. Have you ever seen a balloon take in air and get smaller, then give off air and get bigger?

Stop and think for a moment about your own breathing. Is it closer to the proper or improper methods just described?

Deep Abdominal Breathing

This is a concept that while often lauded, is just as frequently misunderstood. When most people hear deep abdominal breathing, their assumption is that they should breathe through their abdominal area alone. This is both untrue and unwise. Your lungs extend from your diaphragm to just above your collarbone. Remember our balloon analogy? Has anyone ever heard of filling only the bottom of a balloon? With each breath make sure to fill your lungs completely in order to get maximum benefit from the 20,000 breaths you will take today.

Forward Breathing

Most people picture their lungs as being located in the front part of their body. In reality, the lungs lie behind the protection of the ribcage, and extend much farther back than is often realized. Because of this, it is common to breathe into the front portion of your lungs, causing breathing to be shallow.

Mouth Breathing

Many people breathe through their mouths. This is especially common for those suffering from respiratory illness, since it is sometimes hard to get enough air into the lungs using the nose alone. The problem with mouth breathing is that your nose is unable to help warm or cool the air you take in, or to filter out impurities. When breathing through your nose, particles in the air are removed by tiny hairs inside your nostrils, as well as bony ridges located inside your nasal cavities. As a result, mouth breathing should be kept to a minimum, particularly in extremely hot, cold or polluted environments.

Accessory Breathing

Accessory breathing is performed using neck, shoulder and chest muscles. This places tremendous pressure on the jaw, cervical spine and vocal chords. According to breathing coordination instructor, Jessica Wolf, blowing out your vocal chords is a common result of accessory breathing.

Tight Clothes

From corsets to jeans that fit like a second skin, tight clothing has long been the enemy of proper breathing. I'm by no means free of guilt. I tend to wear my pants pretty tight (I'm still a size 30, darn it!).

The reality is that this type of clothing restricts, and therefore impairs normal respiratory function.

Smoking

When listing the factors that impair your ability to breathe normally there is no bigger culprit than smoking. It is a primary cause of lung cancer, emphysema and numerous other types of respiratory illness, as well as heart disease and strokes. Worldwide, approximately five million people die from tobacco-related diseases annually with over 400,000 of those in the US and another 45,000 in Canada. It is estimated that regular tobacco use cuts approximately fifteen years off each smoker's life.

Asthma

Over 20 million Americans suffer from asthma, a serious condition involving the inflammation of the airways. Should a substance to which the asthmatic is sensitive provoke a reaction, their airways may further swell, making breathing difficult. This can result in wheezing, coughing, chest tightness, and trouble breathing. Both the severity and duration of such attacks vary widely. Should an attack be prolonged or severe, a medical emergency may ensue. Unless dealt with properly, these situations can be life-threatening.

Numerous substances can provoke an asthma attack. They include, smoke, dust mites, pollen, cold air and animal dander. Stress is also a factor, making effective stress-management a key to avoiding future attacks.

Asthma is a condition that can be controlled. Medication is helpful, but prevention is key. By identifying, then avoiding those substances to which the asthmatic is sensitive, attacks can be prevented and a normal life can be led.

Solutions

Exercises

*Slow Your Breathing: Many people breathe too rapidly and rapid breathing tends to be shallow. Try counting as you breathe. After you get the sequence, cut it in half, making each inhalation and exhalation last twice as long.

*Reverse Your Breathing: For those who breathe paradoxically, this exercise can help. Lie on your back with a pillow on your stomach. As you inhale watch to see that the pillow rises. If it does, then your inhalation is falling in the proper place within the breathing cycle. Remember: inhale, pillow rises, exhale, pillow falls.

*Combination: Here is an exercise that I find helpful in developing proper breathing habits. Start by sitting comfortably and folding your arms gently over your ribcage, with your fingers spread wide. Next, as you slowly begin to inhale, feel your ribs as they expand against your arms, then gradually open your arms wide as air continues to fill your lungs. After inhaling, fully exhale, allowing your arms to slowly move back to their starting position. Each inhalation and exhalation should take several seconds. If as you inhale you feel your ribcage move away from your arms instead of pressing against them then you are experiencing paradoxical breathing. Since doing this exercise in public might not be practical, master it at home first, then continue to use the imagery once you leave the house. By doing so, you can continue the exercise even when your arms are busy holding a newspaper or controlling your steering wheel.

*Overcome Forward Breathing: As mentioned earlier, many people breathe into the front portion of their lungs. To overcome this tendency, each time you take a breath, focus on filling your back with air. A word of caution, do not allow this to reverse your breathing. As you inhale your lungs should expand both forward and backward, filling the entire balloon with air.

Air Purifiers

How you breathe is important, but so is what you breathe. Whether in your home, office or taking a lap around the track, the air you inhale often contains a number of potentially harmful contaminants. These include dust, mold, smoke, pollen and animal dander, just to name a few. There are many products currently available that promise to solve this problem for you. They range from decorative lamps made of Himalayan salt that can be had for as little as $20, to large machines costing $700 or more. There are also small, portable devices that can be used to cleanse the air in your car or hotel room.

The question is do any of these products make a *real* difference in air quality? According to *Consumer Reports* the results are iffy at best. Their research found that some of the best known brands were unable to clean the air to any meaningful degree. In addition, machines that give off a significant amount of ozone can be harmful to asthmatics and impair normal lung function in the rest of the population.

Since there is little hard evidence to support the value of these devices, I suggest thinking twice before plunking down a week's pay for something that might do more harm than good. If you do decide to invest in such an item, most of the data I've seen suggests getting one that emits negative ions. In that case even if it doesn't help, hopefully it also won't hurt.

Breathing Coordination

This is a system that was developed in the 1950s, by vocal instructor Carl Stough, who found it effective in alleviating the suffering of emphysema patients. According to instructor Jessica Wolf:

> "The body is designed in a particular way to move air out of and into the lungs. *Breathing Coordination* is the exact way the respiratory system is designed to function at maximum efficiency with minimum effort. The unique aspect of this method is that the coordination is the correct pattern for a particular individual, not a general pattern which can be applied to every individual. It recognizes the individualistic pattern of breathing which distributes the work of breathing equally over the entire respiratory system."

Yoga and Breathing (Pranayama)

In most forms of yoga there is a tremendous emphasis placed on proper breathing. It is common to begin and end classes with five minutes of Yogic breathing, much as a warm-up and a cool down should be included in any exercise routine. According to instructor Anne Taylor, the breathing techniques that yoga employs benefit you by bringing awareness to your physical body as well as calming you and helping you focus. There are many methods to choose from depending on both the individual's personality and situation. In the morning, an invigorating technique like Breath of Fire could be the correct choice. It is a Kundalini yoga technique that involves breathing fast and hard, using only your nose. In the evening, a calming technique such as Dirgha pranayama, where inhalations are deep and slow, might be more appropriate.

Chi Gung

This method of maintaining one's health and vitality was developed in China over 4500 years ago. One of the key components of Chi Gung is breathing. Exercises incorporate movement patterns with breathing techniques in order to strengthen the inner life force or Chi. The beauty of Chi Gung is its simplicity. Unlike yoga, there are no complex poses. Exercises are easy to do and require no partner or equipment. If you're interested in learning more about Chi Gung read *Ch'I the*

Power Within: Chi Kung Breathing Exercises for Health, Relaxation and Energy by Geoff and Phyllis Pike.

Frog Breathing

This is an adaptive response to the loss of elasticity in the lungs, due to respiratory illness. Glossopharyngeal, or "frog" breathing, involves the gulping of tiny amounts of air until they total the equivalent of a complete breath. While not recommended for the general population, this method can be a blessing for individuals who might otherwise be confined to a breathing machine.

Breathing Tips

*Use the Right Equipment: Remember that proper breathing should engage your ribcage not just your upper chest or stomach. Make sure that each breath is slow and relaxed. Also, allow your back to be involved in the breathing process.

*Start with the Exhale: In order to make room for your next breath, it's necessary to let the air, already in your lungs, out. As Jessica Wolf puts it, "You can't fill a container that's already full."

*Don't Try so Hard: Breathing should be a natural and comfortable process. Ironically, many problems develop when people try too hard to breathe properly.

Suggested Reading

The Art of Breathing: 6 Simple Lessons to Improve Performance, Health, and Well-Being by Nancy Zi (North Atlantic Books, 4th edition, October 30, 2000)

Dr. Breath: The Story of Breathing Coordination by Carl Stough & Reece Stough (Stough Institute, January 1981)

Free Your Breath, Free Your Life: How Conscious Breathing Can Relieve Stress, Increase Vitality, and Help You Live More Fully by Dennis Lewis (Shambhala Publications, Inc. 2004)

Stop Aging or Slow the Process: How Exercise with Oxygen Therapy (EWOT) Can Help by William Campbell Douglass II, MD (Rhino Publishing, S.A., April 2003)

"Rule Number 1 is, don't sweat the small stuff. Rule Number 2 is, it's all small stuff. And if you can't fight and you can't flee, flow."
—Robert S. Eliot

15 | 8:35 a.m. Will you Spend This Time Worrying?

You've just finished practicing your healthy breathing techniques but realize that you're still stressed. Are you thinking about that pile of papers waiting on your desk? Perhaps it's the afternoon meeting for which you're not fully prepared? Your six year old has a birthday party on Saturday and the clown just called in sick? The other chapters in this book discuss things you should consider doing. This chapter is about something that you shouldn't do —Worry.

The Problem

In our society, we are trained to worry. If you don't worry it's as if you don't care. This belief fills us with anxiety that is damaging both physically and mentally. How many of us have had headaches, stomach problems, neck or back pain that was quite real as a result of things that upset us emotionally? Ever hear of a tension headache or a nervous stomach? The relationship between stress and illness is undeniable and has been verified by reams of scientific evidence. Worry creates stress and is responsible for many serious health problems including high blood pressure, heart attacks, ulcers and breakdown of the immune system.

Solutions

Adjust Your Thinking

Don't Make Things Bigger Than They Are

> *"...making a mountain out of a molehill."*
> **—Wilkie Collins**

Is your stomach tied in knots because your favorite baseball team may not win the pennant when not one of their players even knows who you are?

Are you worried because you might have forgotten to tape tonight's Law And Order marathon filled with episodes that you've already seen eight or nine times?

Are you agonizing because your son taught the parrot Spanish and since you don't speak the language you can't tell if it's cursing?

If you answered yes to any of the previous questions or would to others in a similar vein, then it's entirely possible that you're taking the bumps in your road a little too seriously.

One of the reasons people worry is that they see problems as being bigger than they are. One solution is to acknowledge just how small life's daily trials and tribulations really are in the greater scheme of things. This is often easier said than done. Still, by moving in that direction, even one baby step at a time, you may come to realize that your situation is far better than you perceive it to be.

Acknowledge That Worry Doesn't Help

> *"God grant us the serenity to accept the things we*
> *cannot change, courage to change the things we*
> *can, and wisdom to know the difference."*
> **—Unknown**

It is important to accept that worry doesn't change anything. You can worry to your heart's discontent about the traffic jam in which you are trapped but that won't get those other cars moving any sooner. On the other hand, by taking the initiative to map out a new route, you might be able to avoid the situation entirely. Once you internalize this concept you can act effectively to alter those situations that you have the power to change and accept those over which you have no control.

Realize that You're Not the Focus

Many people are under the impression that their actions are being closely observed. Whether it's their friends, classmates or the guy seated next to them at the Stones concert, they feel that every blunder, no matter how small, is seen, heard, then debated ad nauseam by all those within eye or earshot. In reality, most people are way too involved in their own lives to dwell on the missteps of yours. The bad news is you may not be as important as you think you are. The good news is nobody cares how badly you danced at the Christmas party, so stop worrying!

Accept that You're Not Alone

One of the problems that a worrier faces is the misguided belief that their fear is unique. Believing that others don't react as *they* do makes the worrier feel weak and inferior. The good news is that you are not alone. No matter how foolish your particular concern seems to be, there are plenty of other people who worry about it, too. Knowing this gives you one less thing to worry about.

Adjust Your Behavior

Worry Less and Do More!

One of the problems with worry is that it shuts down the very creative processes you will need to solve the problems that are troubling you. This creates a cycle that can be difficult to break. The best solution is to take an active role. Below are ten typical examples of debilitating worry along with a simple course of action that could help empower you:

Problem: I'm afraid that my ineffective co-op board may bankrupt the corporation.

Solution: Run for office in the next election. If you win, you will be privy to all decisions made that will effect your investment. If you lose, you will have taken action, which is very empowering. In either case, you will get to know your neighbors.

Problem: I'm overweight and I'm afraid it will ruin my health.

Solution: Begin a diet and exercise routine. This will not only enable you to improve your health, but the endorphins that exercise stirs up will improve your state-of-mind.

Problem: I have to take the subway home from work at night through a dangerous area.

Solution: Take a self-defense course. This will prepare you both physically and mentally to deal with trouble, should it arise.

Problem: I read that many vitamins don't contain the ingredients that they advertise. Are the vitamins I paid so much for really helping me?

Solution: Refer to chapter eight for websites that can give you valuable information on the validity of supplements then use your computer to do some research.

Problem: If I don't quit smoking, I'm going to die!

Solution: See a specialist. There are many qualified therapists who specialize in helping those addicted to tobacco to kick the habit. Perhaps you prefer to handle things yourself. One option is to cut down gradually. Try putting yourself on a "smoking schedule". If you currently smoke 20 cigarettes per day, smoke 19 tomorrow, then reduce your total by one each day until you are smoke-free.

Problem: I'm never going to be able to support my family on the money I'm making.

Solution: Ask your boss for a raise. Another option is looking for a higher paying job. Perhaps one appeals to you for which you are not qualified. In that case, consider going back to school. This will enable you to work towards your goal.

Problem: When I retire, will my pension enable me to live comfortably?

Solution: Meet with a financial advisor. They make a living addressing the type of concerns that are causing you sleepless nights. A plan can be set up to make the extra years this book is helping you to live as happy as they are healthy.

Problem: Does the person I'm interested in dating share my feelings?

Solution: You'll never know unless you ask. Even if it doesn't work out, taking control of the situation may make you feel empowered. This is a stark contrast to the powerless way you will feel when you just stand around waiting for something to happen.

Problem: Will the new neighbors upstairs blast their TV again like they did last night?

Solution: Try talking to them. You'll be surprised how cooperative people can be. First, introduce yourself and welcome them to the building, then bring up the problem. If that doesn't work, speak to the building manager and find out what the noise regulations are, then take appropriate action.

Problem: I just read a report on prostate cancer that frightened me. Am I at risk?

Solution: See your doctor. A simple blood test, called a PSA test can indicate if you are at risk. Taken annually it can set your mind at ease. If by chance the unthinkable is found, early detection makes prostate cancer highly curable.

Can't Keep your Schedule Straight?

This is a problem many people face. Below are some general solutions that can help organize your time and clear your head.

Buy a Calendar

Writing your appointments on a wall calendar will stop you from struggling to keep them straight in your head. Make sure it's one that you like. Whether its cute puppies or race cars, it's important that your calendar has pictures that you find appealing. That way you will look forward to the experience on a subconscious level, making it more likely that it will become habit.

Don't Worry, Be Techie

Electronic Organizers: The age of technology has taken a bad rap, sometimes deservedly so. Still, when it comes to getting yourself organized, it offers some options that are hard to beat. If it's challenging for you to remember everything on your busy schedule consider purchasing an electronic organizer. Prices range from under twenty dollars for a simple electronic personal organizer to three hundred dollars for a Palm Pilot. They make it easy to get your life in order so that you can worry about it less. One model that costs $19.99 even offers an English-Spanish translator so that the next time Montezuma's revenge kicks in you won't have to worry about how to ask where the bathroom is, not to mention keeping tabs on that darn parrot!

Personal Computer: Your friendly PC can be a big help. By setting it to remind you of important items on your schedule, you will never miss another haircut or doctor's appointment. Multiple reminders are also an option. For example, your computer can be set to remind you a week before, a day before and an hour before your appointment so whether it's a hot date or dinner with your in-laws, you'll never keep them waiting again.

Cell Phone: If you're not near your computer, your cell phone can also help you out. It can be set to beep, then flash the information you're concerned about remembering. Many offer reminders ranging from five minutes to one week before the event in question.

Suggested Reading

Don't Sweat the Small Stuff--and it's all small stuff by Richard Carlson (Hyperion, January 1, 1997)

A Don't Sweat the Small Stuff Treasury: A Special Collection for the Office (Don't Sweat the Small Stuff) by Richard Carlson (Hyperion, Miniature edition, April 5, 2000)

The Worry Cure by Robert L. Leahy (Harmony, November 1, 2005)

CD or Cassette

21 Ways to Stop Worrying by Albert Ellis Ph.D.

"A book holds a house of gold."
—A Chinese Proverb

"Knowledge is wealth that can't be stolen."
—A Philippine Proverb

16 | 8:40 a.m.
Will You Learn
Something New?

Not long ago I ran into one of my elderly neighbors as she pulled one of those little suitcases on wheels through our building's lobby. As we exchanged pleasantries she told me she was coming from her painting class. This was a woman in her eighties, a cancer survivor with a hip replacement, conditions that would turn many people into couch potatoes. Still, it wasn't keeping her from enjoying her retirement by expanding her mind and learning something new. Ever hear the expression, "You can't teach old dog new tricks"? Well who wants to be an old dog anyway? Learning is one of the things that keep us young.

In their book, *Living to 100: Lessons in Living to Your Maximum Potential at Any Age*, Thomas T. Perls, M.D. and Margery Hutter Silver, Ed.D., point out the role that keeping an active mind has played in the lives of those who have reached the magic one hundred year plateau. They showed how many centenarians still worked, baked and exercised at an age where most Americans had long since given up such activities. In addition, Emma Shulman of NYU Medical Center's Silberstein Institute for Aging and Dementia, credits a greater willingness to learn new things as one of the reasons why women tend to live longer than men. "When they retire, they enroll in classes and are constantly learning," points out Ms. Shulman, herself 93 years young.

The Effects of an Active Mind

Exercising your mind does more than keep your morale up. Science has proven that the more you use your brain, the more efficiently it works. Our brains have billions of cells, also referred to as neurons. By using your brain in ways that are unfamiliar, new connections can be established between these neurons. These connections help you to develop both new skills and new ideas.

Why not take advantage of your morning commute to expand your knowledge in an exciting new way? If you take a train or a bus, then read a book or magazine. If you drive, then consider popping in an educational tape or CD.

Some Suggestions for After Work

> *"Do not be too timid or squeamish about your actions. All life is an experiment."*
> **—Ralph Waldo Emerson**

While learning something new can be a lively and invigorating experience, everyone's quest for knowledge takes them in a different direction. Here are a few ideas that might expand your horizons in a positive way:

*Learn a New Language: Tired of going to Mexico and feeling like the tourist you are? Want to be able to chat with the Chinese family next door? Wonder if your Korean manicurist is gossiping about you? (Yes, I watch *Seinfeld*). Learning a new language is both a practical skill to have and a mind expanding experience.

*Study a Musical Instrument: As a drummer, I'm well aware of the thrill that comes from expressing yourself musically. It's the feeling you get from creating something beautiful where nothing existed just seconds before. But be considerate. Getting punched out by an irate neighbor who didn't enjoy your 3:00 AM tuba concert certainly won't extend your life.

*Take a Computer Class: This is directed primarily at those who have yet to break down and buy a PC so they can geek along with the rest of us. I speak from experience, having held out for several years while all my friends were happily cruising down the information superhighway. I can tell you that once you make the move, there's no turning back. The knowledge available on the Internet and the ease with which it can be acquired is awe-inspiring. But even for those of us who are functional on these machines (Hey, I wrote this book, didn't I?), there is still plenty more to learn should you choose to take the plunge.

*Take a Dance Class: For experienced dancers, learning a new style can be an enjoyable experience, but even if you have two left feet there's no reason why you can't take them in some new and exciting directions. Dance is good exercise (see chapter 26) as well as a great way to meet new people.

*Take a Cooking Class: Is there a type of food you love and would like to make at home? Always wanted to learn how but have hesitated until now? Here's an opportunity to literally go with your gut.

*Real Estate or The Stock Market: Here is something that might not just expand your field of knowledge but could make you a few bucks as well. Not long ago stocks were all the rage, now it is real estate. Both are interesting topics and the knowledge such a class provides might either help you pull the string on a profitable investment or prevent a mistake far more expensive than the class itself.

*Health: There are plenty of classes involving many aspects of holistic health held in a variety of places on a regular basis. Whether the topic is couples massage, Reiki or meditation, the experience can introduce you to both new concepts and likeminded people, either of which will prove stimulating

Where to Go

If any of these topics sound appealing, you might want to stick a toe in the water before diving right in. Some organizations offer one or two night courses. For a nominal fee, they will give you a taste of what a topic has to offer. Some courses last a full term and are more expensive. Others are free.

*The YMCA: Since its founding in the mid-nineteenth century, the Y has been a resource for adults looking to expand their knowledge in a vast array of topics. Since each Y has different programs to offer, it pays to check with the Y in your area. For general info visit their national website at: www.ymca.net.

*High Schools: Once the kids have gone home, many high schools offer courses to adults in the community. Subject matter often includes courses in English for recent immigrants and computers for those wishing to bring their technological skills up to speed. Check with your local school to find out what courses are available.

*Colleges: Many colleges offer adult education courses. Check and see if one in your area has a class in a subject that interests you.

*The American Red Cross: If you would like to learn first aid, CPR or the skills necessary to become a life guard or child care provider, your local Red Cross offers courses that may be right for you. Visit there website at: www.redcross.org.

*The Library: Libraries around the country offer courses in a variety of subject areas. Contact your local branch for more information.

*The Learning Annex: The Learning Annex has something for everyone. With branches throughout the US and Canada, It offers courses in everything from graphic arts to palm reading. To learn if they have a branch near you, visit their website at: www.learningannex.com.

*The Open Center: A New York based bastion of holistic health courses. Similar organizations exist in cities nationwide. Visit the Open Center's website at: www.opencenter.org.

Want More Info?

The Adult Education Quarterly is a journal that strives to advance the understanding and practice of adult education. You can learn more by visiting their website at: aeq.sagepub.com.

"The trick is growing up without growing old."
—*Casey Stengel*

Section II:

THE WORK DAY

"It's a VERY short trip. While alive, LIVE!"
—Malcolm Forbes

"One of the major reasons why people are not doing well is because they keep trying to get through the day. A more worthy challenge is to try to get from the day."
—Jim Rohn

"We must not allow the clock and the calendar to blind us to the fact that each moment of life is a miracle and mystery."
—H. G. Wells

17 | 9 a.m.
Are You Wishing Your Life Away?

It's nine o'clock and you've just arrived at the office after a particularly grueling commute. You look at your desk and it's piled high with papers. You don't even have your coat off and your phone is lit up, not one line but two. You have a full eight hours of hell staring you in the face and it's not a pretty sight. All you can think of is how you can't wait until it's over, not just the day, but the week. Hey, why stop there? You have a vacation coming at the end of the month. Just think of that beach in Aruba, if you can just get through these next three weeks…At this point I have one piece of advice for you: Stop Wishing Your Life Away! We all do it. "I can't wait until this day is over," "I can't wait until my vacation," and "I can't wait until this pimple on my forehead goes away." It's natural to look forward to the future, but it shouldn't be done at the expense of the present. Life is precious and far too short. If you wish it away that's just where it will go—away. It's a mindset that will make you old before your time.

Refocus

In order to adopt this new attitude you'll need to change your approach a bit. Every set of circumstances can be viewed at least two different ways. Focus on whatever is good about your situation. Is it challenging? Interesting? Or will it just make the future seem better by comparison? Every experience has value even if it's just learning not to have that experience again.

Changing Your Behavior

How often each day do you check your watch? If you're like me, the temptation is always there, even when there is no place in particular you need to go. Think a minute, are you really in that much of a hurry? We've all seen *Seinfeld*. Think of Kramer. He didn't even own a watch. Did he seem stressed out to you?

Does Traffic Make You Crazy?

No one likes sitting in traffic, an experience we've all had at one time or another. Still, how you handle your frustration can add years to your life or subtract them just as easily. A traffic jam is a situation over which you have little control, and people like to feel in control. However, the problem is largely a matter of perception. While your external environment may be out of your hands the internal environment of your vehicle is something you *can* control. This is a place where technology can help. Devices like CD players and satellite radio receivers can help take the sting out of the experience. Try listening to an educational audio tape or CD as was suggested in the previous section. Feeling that your time is not going to waste will go a long way towards making this type of experience more tolerable. Consider hanging something with a pleasant scent inside your car. As you recall from the section on aromatherapy, a fragrance that you enjoy can help ease your frustration and improve your mood.

Waiting in Line

I was waiting in line at the bank on a stiflingly hot July afternoon when in walked one of my elderly neighbors. For whatever reason only one teller was working, causing the line, made up of only six people, to move at a snail's pace. The woman quickly became impatient and began expressing her displeasure to anyone within earshot. In reality, the wait would be no more than fifteen minutes. Was this retiree who lived alone in *that* big of a hurry to leave this air-conditioned bank and reenter the 90 degree heat? Were the few extra minutes she was forced to wait really worth upsetting herself and everyone around her? Did it make the line move any faster?

Suggested Reading

Present Moment Awareness: A Simple, Step-by-Step Guide to Living in the Now by Shannon Duncan (New World Library, April 2003)

The Power of Now: A Guide to Spiritual Enlightenment by Eckhart Tolle (New World Library, Reprint edition, September, 2004

"An apple a day keeps the doctor away."
—A Welsh Folk Proverb

18 | 10 a.m.
Will You Have a
Midmorning Snack?

At this point in the day, it's wise to have a little something to keep those metabolic fires burning. Growing up I always heard how bad it was to snack between meals. We now know that whether it's good or bad depends on what that snack is and how much of it we eat. Since five smaller meals a day are recommended by most health and fitness professionals, a healthful snack at this time of the morning can be a positive thing.

Some Good Choices

Yogurt

Low fat yogurt is a great source of calcium. The types of bacterial cultures yogurt contains can help strengthen your immune system and also do wonders for your digestive tract. Before you buy yogurt, check for the Live and Active Cultures (LAC) seal. Issued by the National Yogurt Association (NYA), this shows that the product contains at least 100 million cultures per gram at the time of manufacture. For extra flavor and health benefit try adding some fresh fruit like blueberries or raspberries.

Nuts

The health benefits that nuts provide have been well documented. Studies have shown that you can lower your risk of cardiovascular disease between 15 and 50 percent by eating just a handful of nuts five times a week. Nuts are also an excellent source of vitamin E, a powerful antioxidant. Good choices include:

A half cup of walnuts: Walnuts have been shown to fight heart disease by raising your level of HDL. They are also rich in the antioxidant glutathione.

A half cup of almonds: These tasty little kernels lower cholesterol and reduce the risk of prostate cancer.

Several Brazil nuts: Brazil nuts are high in the key antioxidant selenium which strengthens the immune system and helps fight cancer. They are also a great source of thiamin.

Seeds

Pumpkin: Long a fixture in many folk remedies, pumpkin seeds are now being taken seriously by the medical community. They contain a wealth of essential minerals including; magnesium, iron, copper and phosphorous. They have also shown promise in combating a number of serious health conditions including heart disease, prostate cancer and arteriosclerosis.

Sunflower: Contain high levels of two key antioxidants, vitamin E and selenium, as well as an assortment of B vitamins and several important minerals. The type of vegetable protein found in sunflower seeds may be effective in combating high blood pressure.

Keep in mind, when it comes to seeds and nuts its way too easy to eat way too many. They taste good and are good for you but have plenty of calories. Because of this, it is recommended that you limit your intake of these snacks to 1-2 oz. per day.

Whole Wheat Pita

These Frisbee like snacks contain no cholesterol or saturated fat and are rich in selenium. They are also high in insoluble fiber, a key weapon in the battle against colon cancer.

Rice Cakes

They don't have much flavor and look like coasters, but when snack time rolls around rice cakes are an excellent choice. They are filling, low in calories and many brands are high in fiber. Go with the whole grain variety whenever possible.

Fruit

Fruit is loaded with heart friendly soluble fiber and cancer fighting antioxidants. Here are some great choices:

Cantaloupe: Some sources consider cantaloupe to be the most nutritious fruit of all. It is rich in both vitamins A and C, and is filled with a high concentration of digestive enzymes. Cantaloupe also contains a substance called myoinositol that is believed to be a weapon in the battle against insomnia, anxiety and arteriosclerosis.

Bananas: There are several reasons why this tasty fruit is an ally in the anti-aging battle. The vitamin B6 that a banana contains helps to prevent insomnia. They also contain the amino acid tryptophan, a precursor of serotonin. Research has shown that elevated serotonin levels help keep depression at bay. Bananas are high in potassium yet low in sodium, a combination that is helpful in preventing strokes. They also contain significant quantities of vitamin C, magnesium and fiber.

Apples: A great source of potassium and both soluble and insoluble fiber. Apples that are not organically grown are often waxed, making peeling a smart choice. If you buy organically grown apples then eat the skin. Much of the vitamin C is located just beneath the skin which also contains lots of insoluble fiber.

Oranges: A rich source of vitamin C, folic acid, potassium and magnesium. Peel but eat the pith between the rind and fruit. It is filled with bioflavonoids which improve the body's utilization of vitamin C.

Grapefruit: Grapefruit is rich in pectin, a type of soluble fiber. This substance has demonstrated the ability to improve glucose tolerance and reduce both blood pressure and levels of LDL. Pink and red grapefruit are high in lycopene, a substance with antioxidant properties. Lycopene helps to keep skin from aging by countering the damaging effects of ultraviolet light, is believed to have the ability to shrink tumors and reduces the risk of macular degeneration.

Grapes (Red and Purple): The synergy of 20 different antioxidants enables grapes to fight aging in a way that no pill can. There is a great deal of evidence to support the cancer fighting properties of both red and purple grapes. Research has shown that both contain chemicals that keep cancer cells from spreading. Keep in mind that the growers of grapes use pesticides quite freely, making the purchase of organically grown grapes an option worth considering.

Strawberries: These sweet red berries are high in vitamin C, calcium, phosphorous and potassium. They also contain compounds called salycilates that are natural pain killers and ellagic acid, a substance that has demonstrated antioxidant properties.

Veggies

Vegetables are packed with vitamins and minerals and should make up a high percentage of our diet. They are a key weapon in the fight against colon cancer, the second deadliest form of the disease in America today. Vegetables, like fruit, are high in both antioxidants and fiber and low in fat. Here are some good choices:

Carrots: Carrots decrease your risk of developing cancer. This is due in part to their high concentration of beta carotene, a key antioxidant. Another compound called falcarinol may be of equal importance. Studies have found that this natural pesticide slows the growth of cancer cells.

Celery: High in fiber, vitamin C and potassium. The fact that you burn more calories by eating and digesting celery than the vegetable contains makes it the perfect diet food. An added perk for men: celery is said to cause men's levels of pheromones, compounds thought to attract women, to rise.

Bell Peppers: Whether red, green or yellow, all bell peppers are a great source of both beta carotene and vitamin C. In addition, green peppers block the formation of carcinogenic compounds known as nitrosamines.

Broccoli: A potent cancer fighter that is high in vitamins A and C and is also a great source of calcium. Broccoli, like other cruciferous vegetables, is particularly valuable in fighting colon cancer. This is due in part to its high concentration of sulforaphane, a powerful cancer-fighting antioxidant. Research done at the Harvard School of Public Health in Boston, found that broccoli reduces the risk of developing cataracts or of having a stroke. Broccoli's high chromium content helps raise levels of DHEA, a hormone that helps to slow the aging process.

Cauliflower: The key nutrients that are abundant in cauliflower include selenium, folate and glutathione. This combination helps fight cancer and arteriosclerosis, strengthens the immune system and regulates blood pressure.

Edamame: Literally translated as "beans on branches," edamame are better known as soybeans. They offer a complete protein as well as high concentrations of calcium, vitamin A and several B vitamins.

Sorry To Disappoint You

No matter how the government classifies them, French fries are not on our list of vegetables

Popcorn

While the nutritional value is minimal, if it's junk food you must have, then this is the least of many available evils. Avoid brands with added butter or salt. Tasty as these additives may be the risks posed to both your health and waistline are substantial.

Suggested Reading

Snacking Habits for Healthy Living by American Dietetic Association (Wiley, September 20, 1997)

*"To me luxury is to be at home with my daughter,
and the occasional massage doesn't hurt."*
—Olivia Newton-John

19 Noon
When Was Your
Last Massage?

Most people I know get an hour for lunch. Here's a great way to spend the first 30 minutes:

Shiatsu, Acupressure, Swedish or Rolfing, whatever the style, massage has long been a part of many people's fitness and wellness routines. It has been used for over 3000 years throughout the world to medicate, relax and invigorate. The Encyclopedia Britannica defines massage as, "The systematic and scientific manipulation of body tissues, performed with the hands, for therapeutic effect on the nervous and muscular systems and on systemic circulation".

While there may be as many styles of massage as there are practitioners, in order to get a broader understanding of the subject it's worth taking a look at some of the best known varieties.

Acupressure: Developed in China, this style of massage can correctly be described as acupuncture without the needles. Pressure is used on points in the body called meridians to alleviate blockages that allow toxins to build up, thereby restoring homeostasis.

Shiatsu: Literally translated as finger pressure, Shiatsu is similar in many ways to acupressure. Developed in Japan, it uses pressure from the fingers to rebalance the body's energy thereby positively affecting the life force or "Chi."

Anma: A Japanese word that literally translated means massage. Many believe that Shiatsu sprung from one of Anma's several distinctly different techniques. In addition to more tangible benefits like improving the functioning of one's muscles, Anma's goals include focusing on the internal life force or "Ki."

Swedish Massage: This is the classic Western style of massage. Its development is generally attributed to a Swedish doctor by the name of Per Henrik Ling. Its primary goal is to increase the blood's oxygen flow and release toxins trapped in the muscles. To this end, pressure is applied against the muscles in the same direction as the flow of blood returning to the heart.

Deep Tissue Massage: This style is similar in many ways to Swedish massage but uses pressure that is often far more intense. Its goal is to reach deeper layers of muscle than can be reached by traditional massage and once there, to break up scar tissue that may have formed, thus restoring normal function.

Sports Massage: This is a blend of several other styles that has become increasingly popular. It is used before and after activity to improve performance and prevent injury.

Rolfing: This system of soft tissue manipulation was developed in the 1950s by Dr. Ida P. Rolf. Its proponents claim that it enhances neurological functioning, thereby facilitating a more efficient use of one's muscles. Rolfing can be helpful to those suffering from a number of ailments, including whiplash that often prove resistant to other methods of treatment. On the down side, Rolfing can be more expensive and more painful than most other styles of bodywork and may result in some bruising. Initial treatment, usually consisting of ten one hour sessions, attempts to loosen the connective tissue thereby allowing muscles to move more freely. This is generally followed by periodic "tune ups" with the frequency specific to individual need. For more information about Rolfing and help choosing a practitioner, visit the Rolf Institute of Structural Integration's website at: www.rolf.org.

Thai Massage: Thought to have originated in India some 2500 years ago, Thai massage is one of the four components of the traditional style of medicine practiced in Thailand. Sometimes called the lazy man's yoga, it differs from Western massage in a number of ways. The client receives their treatment while fully dressed, a plus for the more modest among us. Also, Thai massage uses pressing movements rather than the rubbing motions common in Western massage.

Massage Credentials

Today this ancient art is dealing with the complications of western society through licensing requirements that vary state to state. New York and Nebraska's 1000 hours of training are the most stringent while California's are perhaps the most lax. Liability insurance is also a necessity in many areas as are credits in continuing education. A national certification exam now exists and is required by many states.

On the following page are the state requirements for certification as of November 2006. It will give you a sense of how much training the person about to manipulate your body has received. Keep in mind that regulations often change. Checking with your local city or state will let you know what their current requirements are.

As the list on page 122 illustrates, requirements vary widely. While the continuing education credits needed to maintain one's credentials are not included, they range from zero to 18 hours annually. The states not listed either have no requirements or are awaiting the passage of legislation. This means that in those states clients must be especially careful that they are receiving quality care rather than allowing their body to be manipulated by an individual with a slick rap and few qualifications.

In addition to obtaining the certification required in their area, current practitioners are often members of organizations such as the American Massage Therapy Association (AMTA), which boasts 53,000 members in 27 countries. Founded in 1943, the AMTA's stated goal is to advance the art, science and practice of massage therapy. For more information on the AMTA visit their website at: www.amtamassage.org.

Sports and Massage

Today's athlete has come to value the benefits of massage, with many gyms and sports franchises having a massage therapist on staff. It has proven helpful, not only in relieving pain and soreness resulting from physical activity, but also in improving circulation and range of motion. This in turn helps prevent injury, and prepares athletes to perform maximally. Massage also helps speed recovery from delayed onset muscle soreness as well as injury. According to Wendy Barreto, a graduate of the Swedish Institute, massage helps athletes by realigning muscle fibers to help muscles grow in the right direction. Massage is a valuable tool in reducing stress, thereby allowing athletes to focus better. On the scientific front, numerous studies have provided evidence that massage positively alters the body biochemically, decreasing levels of substances that are detrimental to achieving peak performance.

Alabama	650 hours *
Arizona	500 hours *
Arkansas	500 hours, state exam or *
California	Varies County to County
Connecticut	500 hours *
Delaware	500 hours *: Massage therapist, 300 hours *: Massage technician
District of Columbia	500 hours *
Florida	500 hours *
Georgia	500 hours *
Hawaii	570 hours, written state exam
Illinois	500 hours * or other approved exam
Iowa	500 hours *
Kentucky	600 hours * or NCAA approved certifying exam
Louisiana	500 hours * or written and oral exams
Maine	500 hours, CPR and first aid training *
Maryland	Certified massage therapist 500 hours + 60 college credits * or NCCAOM + state exam Registered massage therapist 500 hours * or NCCAOM + state exam
Massachusetts	500 hours
Mississippi	700 hours, CPR and first aid *
Missouri	500 hours *
Nebraska	1,000 hours + practical exam *
Nevada	Hours Of Study To Be Determined *
New Hampshire	750 hours + CPR *
New Jersey	500 hours * or Diploma from a state approved school
New Mexico	650 hours, state exam *
New York	1000 hours, state exam
North Carolina	500 hours *
North Dakota	750 hours, practical exam and state exam*
Ohio	600 hours, state exam
Oregon	500 hours, practical exam *
Rhode Island	500 hours *
South Carolina	500 hours *
South Dakota	500 hours *
Tennessee	500 hours *
Texas	300 hours, written and practical exam
Utah	600 hours, state exam *
Virginia	500 hours *
Washington	500 hours *
West Virginia	500 hours or *
Wisconsin	600 hours, state exam *

*States currently requiring practitioners to pass the national exam (NCBTMB) or its predecessors (NCETMB or NCE.)

No Pain No Gain?

Many people think of massage as a luxurious and sensual experience. Still, anyone who has had one for strictly therapeutic purposes knows it can also be pretty painful at times. Styles like acupressure, deep tissue and Rolfing put pressure, sometimes a substantial amount of pressure, on very sensitive areas of the body in order to restore normal functioning. The good news is that the temporary pain of the massage can produce long lasting pain relief, a trade off that proves more than worthwhile.

Water and Massage

It is believed by many that by loosening the muscles massage releases toxins back into the system. Those poisons then need to be flushed from the body. Drinking water after your session is completed can help make this process more efficient.

Reasons Why a Massage Therapist Might Not Work for You

While receiving a massage can be both a healthy and a pleasurable experience, there are several reasons why going to a massage therapist may not work for you.

- Some people are uncomfortable being touched by strangers. If this is this case and you are unable to overcome this uneasiness you may tense up, defeating the massage's very purpose.

- It is possible that you may not be able to find a therapist in your area. While the relaxation provided by a massage is undeniable, rushing frantically to and from your appointment may leave you with more stress than you started with.

- Massage is expensive, often as much as one hundred dollars an hour. Many therapists offer half hour sessions, making it a bit more affordable.

- It is possible that your schedule is extremely tight and finding time for a massage would be difficult.

If any of those issues are a problem that you cannot resolve there is still another option, to literally take matters into your own hands.

Self-Massage

When it is impractical to visit a therapist, self-massage can also be helpful. Even when working with someone highly qualified, clients are often encouraged to augment their treatment by working on themselves between sessions. A book called *Self-Massage: Therapeutic Techniques to Relax, Soothe and Stimulate Your Body*, written by Monika Struna and Connie Church is an excellent resource for information on this topic. It gives you plenty of practical advice on how to help relieve some of the same problems for which many people visit a therapist. An advantage of self-massage is your ability to feel when you hit the exact spot that is causing the problem. Still, there is no substitute for proper training so self massage works best when supervised by a highly skilled professional.

Massage Tools

Massage oil: This is a standard tool for any massage therapist and comes both scented and unscented.

The Theracane: This is a handy tool for those doing self-massage. It is a hooked stick with several knobs placed along it at various points. Its shape allows you to work on areas that you otherwise could not reach.

Foam Roll: These have become standard equipment in many gyms. By positioning trouble spots over the hard foam surface, adhesions can be broken up and normal functioning restored.

The Shiatsu Hoop: By pulling the ends of this device together small balls attached to it can be positioned over hard to reach areas like the upper trapezius. The hoop's turnbuckle can be adjustable to fit a variety of body types.

The Moon Car: I discovered this item some years ago while attending a holistic health expo with one of my clients. It is basically a plastic roller with some magnets inside that are supposed to add to its therapeutic value. When rolled over various parts of the body it is said to provide relief from nagging injuries.

If you are in the market for massage tools or books an excellent website is: www.bodywork.com.

Speaking of Which: Suggested Reading

Basic Clinical Massage Therapy: Integrating Anatomy and Treatment (Lww Massage Therapy & Bodywork Series) by James H. Clay, David M. Pounds (Lippincott Williams & Wilkins, August 2002)

The Trigger Point Therapy Workbook: Your Self-Treatment Guide for Pain Relief by Clair Davies, et al (New Harbinger Publications; 2nd edition, July 2004)

A Final Thought

In closing it is safe to say that massage, while not a cure-all, has value. If you're an athlete it may help you perform better. If a higher quality of life is your goal, consider including it. In either case it shouldn't be ignored.

Alternative Treatments

Massage can definitely help with a number of ailments, but if your condition is more serious, you might want to consider the following two methods of alternative medicine.

Chiropractic

When looking for a holistic approach that treats a wide variety of ailments, chiropractic is a popular and often effective option. In its purest form, chiropractic is a method of realigning or "adjusting" the spine. This removes impediments to proper nerve flow, and thereby restores normal functioning. Many of today's practitioners also use a variety of high tech equipment to both diagnose and treat a myriad of disorders.

The development of modern chiropractic is attributed to Daniel David Palmer, a healer plying his trade in Iowa during the late 1800s. The discoveries he made led to his founding of The Palmer School of Chiropractic in 1897. His work was later expanded upon by his son B.J. Palmer, who in 1906 purchased the school. Differences in the strong views held by the two practitioners led to a strained relationship that persisted until the death of D.D. Palmer in 1913.

Qualifications

While licensing requirements for chiropractors vary from state to state, a minimum of two years in an undergraduate program containing a full compliment of appropriate science content is generally required. This is followed by four to five years in an accredited chiropractic college. Minimum hours of study should total no less than 4200. Several different organizations cover the many chiropractors working today. Perhaps the best known is the American Chiropractic Association. For more information you can visit their website at: www.amerchiro.org.

Suggested Reading

Chiropractic First by Terry A. Rondberg, D.C. (Chiropractic Journal, January 1996)

Acupuncture

By now, nearly everyone is familiar with this concept of inserting tiny needles into various points on the body in order to treat numerous types of pain or illness. In spite of this, many are yet to experience its benefits.

How It Works

To understand acupuncture you must be aware of the Eastern concept that all things are interrelated as parts of a universal whole. According to this philosophy, when an obstruction arises in one area of the body, it affects all others. It is believed that energy flows through the human body along lines called meridians. Acupuncture is based on the concept that if this energy flow is interfered with, the problem can be eliminated by placing small needles at the point of the obstruction, thus returning the body to a state of balance.

Qualifications

The licensing requirements for acupuncturists vary from state to state, as does the list of ailments that practitioners are permitted to treat.

For more information on acupuncture visit:

www.acupuncture.com

www.medicalacupuncture.org

"You are what you eat."
—A saying first used in the 1960's

20 | 12:30 p.m. What Will You Have For Lunch?

Eating a healthy lunch can be a challenge since most working people don't have the luxury of eating at home. If this is your situation then you have two choices, bring your food with you or buy something. Consider these options:

Bringing Your Lunch

According to Doctor Pentz, "Healthy lunches should include a complex carbohydrate (hopefully whole grain), protein, and a fruit or vegetable. Any combination of these makes for a healthy and complete lunch: Tuna, whole grain bread, fruit; rice, chicken, and broccoli; cottage cheese, fruit, and whole grain crackers, etc."

If you are bringing your lunch then good choices include:

Brown rice and beans: This combo offers a complete protein and lots of fiber. If you use canned beans make sure to rinse them thoroughly to remove excess sodium. To vary the taste, consider adding corn, another excellent source of fiber.

Pasta and broccoli: Another complete protein, loaded with complex carbohydrates plus all the health benefits broccoli has to offer. Use

127

whole wheat pasta whenever possible. When compared with products made from white flour, the whole-wheat variety has approximately three times the fiber and far more vitamins and minerals. Remember to go easy on the spaghetti sauce. Many popular brands contain over 600 milligrams of sodium, more than a quarter of the 2300 milligram per day limit that the U.S. government recommends.

Salad: High in nutritional value and low in calories. If have neither the time nor patience to prepare one for yourself, a company called Ready Pac can help. They offer pre-washed, high quality produce at reasonable prices. While they only sell to retailers, their products are available nationwide. You can contact Ready Pac at 1-800-800-7822 or visit their website: www.ReadyPac.com.

Pita pocket sandwich: A combination of mescaline greens, turkey breast, tomato and onions served in a whole-wheat pita pocket; contains an excellent balance of nutrients.

Natural peanut butter and banana sandwich on whole grain bread: Combines protein, fiber, potassium and heart healthy fats. Remember to choose natural peanut butter over more recognizable brand names that contain heart unfriendly trans fatty acids. Check the label to verify that the brand you choose does not contain artery-clogging substances such as hydrogenated vegetable oils or palm kernel oil.

Eating Out

Salad Bars

Though they can be pricey, few establishments can match the variety of nutrient packed fruits and vegetables that a good salad bar provides. Keep in mind however, when you're dumping all those goodies in the little plastic tray, that it is easy to over order and therefore overeat. Avoid drowning your salad in dressing, which is loaded with calories and high in saturated fat. Finally, make sure the food is fresh. A salad stops being healthy when the strawberries are fuzzy or the lettuce is brown.

Sandwich Shops

If fast food is the direction you end up going, then sandwich shops like Subway offer some good options. Choose sandwiches on either whole wheat or honey oat bread with lean meats like chicken or turkey. Make sure to add plenty of vegetables (tomatoes, peppers, onions, olives, etc.)

If you add dressing, choose oil and vinegar. Another good choice from Subway is their grilled chicken and baby spinach salad. It also allows you to add from a nice selection of vegetables.

Chinese Restaurants

Many people order Chinese food for lunch since it is tasty, cheap and readily available. Still, there are numerous ingredients in many popular dishes that can prove harmful. While it is safe to say that no one will confuse this type of cuisine with health food, by following a few common sense guidelines you can make your dining experience a healthier one.

Hold the MSG: Monosodium Glutamate is a common food additive. Restaurants love MSG because it fools your brain into thinking that food tastes better than it actually does. This allows them to use lesser quality ingredients and still make customers happy. But fooling you into eating lower quality food is not MSG's only offense. Many people are highly allergic to MSG. Common reactions include headaches, asthma attacks and in some cases seizures. Because of this, it is recommended that you ask for your food to be prepared without MSG.

Steamed Instead of Fried: Substitute items like steamed dumplings for fried ones like egg rolls and fried wontons. By doing so, you can reduce your meal's level of saturated fat.

Have Some Vegetables: Vegetables like broccoli and water chestnuts are an integral part of many dishes, yet people opt for others filled with barely recognizable cuts of meat.

Choose Brown Rice: Many restaurants will allow you to substitute brown rice for the fried variety. If the location you dine in does not, and enough people ask for it, they soon will.

Hold the Shark Fin Soup: Many people are put off by the hefty price of this delicacy. For those who are not, there is an even greater concern—shark fins are high in mercury. Since mercury can damage the brain and kidneys, it should be eliminated from your diet whenever possible.

Drink Some Tea: Perhaps the healthiest item in a Chinese restaurant is contained in that ever present tea pot. If you have just finished your meal and have not yet indulged, try a cup. The benefits of tea will be discussed in detail in chapter 30.

Pizza

Americans love pizza. This lunchtime favorite is everywhere you look, with U.S. sales currently topping $30 billion per year. Still, while you're enjoying that slice from your favorite pizzeria, it is important to keep an eye on the calorie count. Depending on the amount of cheese and choice of toppings, a single slice can easily exceed 400 calories, much of that saturated fat. We all want to enjoy a slice from time to time, so here are a few suggestions:

Watch the Cheese: "More cheese on your pizza means more crust in your arteries," says Jayne G. Hurley, senior nutritionist with the Center for Science in the Public Interest. She recommends foregoing popular options such as stuffed crust and double helpings of mozzarella and instead suggests ordering your slice with half the normal amount of cheese.

Veggies, Please: Any pizza lover knows that there are many toppings available. Choose vegetables like spinach or broccoli over fatty meats such as beef and sausage.

Know When to Say When: One slice of pizza won't kill you, but that doesn't mean you should have five. Be aware that pizza not only has a lot of saturated fat but also has loads of sodium so keep your portions reasonable.

Drink Water: Many establishments offer lunch specials that include a soda. If good health is on your agenda, spend the extra money and get yourself a bottle of water.

Condiments: Part of the Problem

The healthiest lunch can be compromised by loading up on condiments that are full of salt, sugar and saturated fat. Below are some of the worst offenders:

Salad Dressing: The fat content and chemicals in many commercial salad dressings can do more harm than the salad does good. Always ask for the dressing on the side, enabling you, not the cook, to control how much you use.

Tomato Sauce: While tomatoes themselves are a great addition to your diet, many brands of tomato sauce are high in sugar and chemical additives.

Soy Sauce: This is a popular condiment in every Chinese restaurant. Unlike soy itself, which is rich in heart healthy isoflavones, this namesake is a poor source of those compounds. Instead, soy sauce is loaded with sodium and a bunch of unhealthy chemicals.

Some Healthy Condiment Options

While condiments are often the enemy of an otherwise healthy midday meal, some are better than others, possibly even turning a minus into a plus. Good choices include:

Hummus: Made from chick peas, hummus is packed with protein, minerals and fiber. Hummus is ideal for spreading on pita bread or rice cakes.

Natural Peanut Butter: High in both vitamins and minerals, peanut butter is also a great source of monounsaturated fats, which are helpful in lowering cholesterol. Great for spreading on whole wheat bread or whatever suits your fancy.

Garlic Powder: A great substitute for salt. Its strong flavor and high nutritional value make garlic powder ideal for those on sodium restricted diets, such as diabetics.

Oil and Vinegar or Apple Cider Vinegar Salad Dressing: While most commercial salad dressings are loaded with saturated fats, these options offer a healthy assortment of monounsaturated and polyunsaturated fatty acids.

Lunchtime Pitfalls

*Soda: Drinking sugar-sweetened soft drinks on a daily basis drastically increases your risk of obesity and the development of type II diabetes. As for diet soda, while the calorie count may be low, the artificial sweeteners it contains can cause a wide variety of ailments. Perhaps the worst offender is aspartame, an ingredient in most diet sodas. Aspartame intake has been linked to over 90 different symptoms including headaches, nausea, depression, memory loss and heart palpitations. It is believed that frequent intake of aspartame can lead to serious health problems such as blindness, seizures or chronic pain. There is also mounting evidence that drinking carbonated beverages, such as soda robs your body of calcium, thus putting you at greater risk for osteoporosis. Soda also promotes tooth decay.

*Ordering "The Meal": Many restaurants offer a lunch combo. They do so to please customers whose appetites are bigger than their wallets.

The problem is that when given the opportunity, many people will clean their plates — all of them. According to dietician Linda Feingold, this is a marketing ploy to which we should all grow wise, "You shouldn't have to make a choice between saving calories and saving money," states Ms. Feingold, "Order foods a la carte."

*Hold the Fries: Fried foods are a killer and this lunchtime favorite is no exception. A king-sized order of fries from one national fast food chain weighs in at an astounding 600 calories. That same bag of fries also contains 75 percent of your daily allotment of artery clogging saturated fat.

*Desserts (Donuts, Cake, Ice Cream, etc): Adding these to an otherwise healthy meal can tip the scales against you and fast. The refined sugar in treats like these is largely responsible for America's ever expanding waistline as well as our high levels of type II diabetes, heart disease and high blood pressure. Many desserts also contain trans fats and a variety of chemicals. Trans fats, often used as a preservative, are a known carcinogen.

Suggested Reading

Restaurant Confidential by Michael F. Jacobson and Jayne Hurley (Workman Publishing Company, May 6, 2002)

"Health, a light body, freedom from cravings, a glowing skin, sonorous voice, fragrance of body: these signs indicate progress in the practice of meditation."
—Shvetashvatara Upanishad

"Meditation is the tongue of the soul and the language of our spirit."
—Jeremy Taylor

21 Somewhere Between 3 p.m. and 5:30 p.m. Will You Meditate Again?

Meditating twice a day is highly recommended. In some ways, the second meditation is more important than the first. If you run a machine continually it will eventually break down. Your body is no different. This brief respite allows you to recharge, much as the siesta has in Portugal, Spain and Latin America for hundreds of years. If you can find a quiet place in the mid to late afternoon, do it then. If you take mass transit home then the ride is also an excellent time for session number two. In either case, try to work both meditations into your schedule. I think you'll find the results well worth the effort.

Tips

Some elements that were easily controllable during meditation number one may be less so here, especially if session two is done in public. Below are several factors mentioned the first time around that might now present more of a challenge. Remember not to fret too much about them. The main thing is that you get both meditations in.

*Tight Clothes: Since you may be dressed for work, this can be an issue. Whenever possible loosen your belt and/or tie. Kicking off your shoes is also a good idea, assuming you're not in a setting where you're likely to wake up without them.

*Noise: This can be a distraction and when in public, not one you can control. If several settings are available then choose the quietest one. Ear plugs are another option. Just make sure you're somewhere safe, since having you're eyes closed and your ears plugged makes you somewhat vulnerable.

*Eating: Remember, whenever possible, to wait at least an hour after eating before beginning a meditation. This will enable you to fully benefit from the experience.

*Cell phones: Few experiences are as distracting as the sudden ring of a phone emanating from your pocket or purse. Even when set on vibrate they can interfere with a mediator's purpose. For this reason, it is best to turn your phone off before beginning to meditate.

"Laugh and your life will be lengthened for this is the great secret of long life."
—Og Mandino

"A person without a sense of humor is like a wagon without springs. It's jolted by every pebble on the road."
—Henry Ward Beecher

22 | 4:55 p.m. Will You Laugh?

On September 18, 2005 the *New York Post* ran a story about a very special man. His name was Arthur Warmington, a native of Morristown, New Jersey. The reason for the story was an event held the previous Friday, or more accurately, the purpose of that event. On that occasion friends and family had gathered at the Masonic Home of New Jersey, in the township of Burlington, to celebrate the birthday of Mr. Warmington, a man they all knew and loved. That alone might not sound like much of a story, except that on that day Arthur Warmington was 110 years old. When asked what his secret was the one thing he could come up with was his cheerful sense of humor. As you near the end of your work day ask yourself, in the past eight hours did you have a good laugh?

Stories such as the one above amuse us, but not all evidence for the benefits of laughter is anecdotal. Studies have shown that those who laugh more often have a significantly reduced risk of developing heart disease, feel less stressed and are better able to tolerate pain. Those are just a few of the ailments for which laughter has proven beneficial.

The Therapeutic Value of Humor

"The art of medicine consists of amusing the patient while nature cures the disease."
—Voltaire

Research has shown humor to be a valuable tool both as preventive medicine and as a method of pain management. It has been found to reduce stress, lower blood pressure and provide a boost to both brain function and the immune system.

- The University of Nebraska reports: "Laughter is very powerful medicine. It can lower stress, dissolve anger and unite families in their resolve to overcome troubled times."

- Researchers at Southern California's Loma Linda University found that watching comedies raised the levels of both endorphins (27 percent) and human growth hormones (87 percent) in healthy test subjects as compared to a control group

- Cardiologists at the University of Maryland Medical Center found that one's sense of humor played a significant role in preventing heart disease

Patch Adams

To see how healthcare and humor can work hand in hand you need look no further than the work of Hunter (Patch) Adams, MD. A brilliant physician, Adams believed in treating the individual as a person, not just a patient. He embraced holistic health methods, shunned by many in the medical community, and used humor to lift the spirits of the sick and injured.

In 1972 Adams founded the Gesundheit! Institute, located in Hillsboro, West Virginia, a unique institution that has treated thousands of patients employing both traditional and alternative styles of medicine. Adams is the author of *Gesundheit!*, a book that describes his work as well as his beliefs about the healthcare system. He was also the subject of the film *Patch Adams*, starring Robin Williams. To learn more about the Gesundheit! Institute, visit their website at: www.PatchAdams.com.

How Humor Saved Norman Cousins

"Humor is mankind's greatest blessing."
—Mark Twain

In 1964, Norman Cousins, a well known writer, was stricken by ankylosing spondylitis, a potentially fatal disease which causes the body's connective tissue to break down. Doctors informed him that his chances of recovery were less than one percent. They gave him only six months to live. Cousins, unwilling to surrender, took matters into his own hands. After leaving the hospital he checked into a hotel. He stopped taking the medication they had prescribed and instead substituted large doses of vitamin C to boost his immune system. He also watched Marx Brothers movies to raise his spirits. Cousins lived until 1990, an additional 26 years. For the rest of his life he attributed the positive feelings those films created as a major factor in his making a full recovery. Cousins life was portrayed in the 1984 film, *Anatomy of an Illness*, starring Edward Asner.

Laughter Clubs

"Laugh and the world laughs with you, weep and you weep alone."
—From the poem Solitude by Ella Wheeler Wilcox

It had long been accepted that laughter was contagious when a Bombay physician by the name of Dr. Madan Kataria found a way to use that fact to the benefit of those around him. In 1995 he formed the first laughter club. Each day Bombay residents would gather in the park to tell jokes and laugh together. Since some jokes were found offensive they soon decided to go straight to the laughter. Participants reported improvements in their health, self confidence and interpersonal relationships and news of the phenomenon spread rapidly. Today there are over 5000 laughing clubs in 53 countries. For information on joining or forming a laughter club in your area: www.worldlaughtertour.com.

The Power of a Smile

"A smile will gain you ten more years of life."
—Chinese Proverb

Few things are as powerful as a smile. A smile on your face makes people like you and feeling appreciated adds years to your life. When you smile, others feel good. What do most sane people do when smiled at? Smile back, of course. It's the gift that keeps on giving. One of the things small town folks complain about when visiting a big city is the unfriendliness of those around them. In reality, they haven't even met 99.9 percent of them, but are judging them solely on their appearance, largely their reluctance to smile at strangers.

An Exercise or Two

Here are a couple of exercises recommended by experts in the field of interpersonal skills. Try them for a week and see how they change the way you feel and how others feel about you.

- In his classic *How to Win Friends & Influence People*, Dale Carnegie suggests smiling at someone every hour for one week

- In His Book *Giant Steps*, Anthony Robbins recommends taking a week and spending one minute, five times a day, standing in front of a mirror grinning

Both of these exercises, while they may seem silly at first, can change the way you feel as well as the mood you project. Why not give them a try?

Find the Humor in the Situation

> *"I think the next best thing to solving a problem is finding some humor in it".*
> —**Frank A. Clark**

When things go wrong, especially in a stressful work environment, this can be easier said than done. There is an old saying that goes, "If life gives you lemons, make lemonade." One of the best examples I can think of occurred in the winter of 2000. My father had developed prostate cancer, and once a month I had to take him to the urologist for a Lupron shot to slow the progress of the disease. He was pretty shaky on his feet, and I had to carefully guide him wherever we went. On this occasion the ground was pretty icy and though we were careful, he slipped and fell flat on his back. I was pretty shook up; after all he was pushing 80 and not in good health. I looked down at him and to my surprise he was laughing heartily. I asked him what could possibly be funny about a situation like this, to which he responded, "You should see the look on your face." I learned something from my father that day. I took him for his shot and we went to lunch.

Suggested Reading

Anatomy of an Illness as Perceived by the Patient by Norman Cousins (W. W. Norton & Company; Reprint edition, July 11, 2005)

Laughter the Best Medicine: The Healing Powers of Happiness, Humour and Joy! by Robert Holden (Thorsons, March 25, 1999)

The Humor Connection, published quarterly by The Association for Applied and Therapeutic Humor (AATH.)

Want More Info?

Looking for more information on the therapeutic value of humor? Funny you should ask:

The Association for Applied and Therapeutic Humor has an excellent website. Visit them at: www.aath.org.

The American Chronic Pain Association dedicates a section of its website to the heading "Inspiration and Humor." You can find it at: http://www.theacpa.org/people/helpful_reading.asp.

Cancer survivors Roger and Kathy Cawthon have a website called: The Cancer Crusade "Fighting cancer with hope and humor." It has a wealth of valuable information and can be found at: www.thecancercrusade.com.

"Watch out for the dangers of an excessive activity, whatever... the job that you hold, because many jobs often lead to the 'hardening of the heart,' as well as 'suffering of the spirit, loss of intelligence.' "
—Saint Bernard

"For we brought nothing into the world, and we certainly can't carry anything out."
-From Paul's first letter to Timothy (I Tim 6:7)

"All work and no play make Jack a dull boy."
—James Howell

---

23 | 5 p.m.
How Many Hours Will You Work?

During the late nineties when I was working as a trainer at an upscale gym in midtown Manhattan, I would marvel at the stressful way many of my clients chose to live. They rose early, and started their day with a long commute in from the suburbs. They worked feverishly all day, often eating a quick lunch at their desk, then raced during a break to the nearest gym. They did so hoping that a short time spent with me would undo all the damage that their stressful lifestyle inflicted upon them. They often came in tense yet tried to minimize the warm-up and stretching components of their workout, a practice that I strongly discouraged. I found this ironic since they were the type of client who needed them the most.

Afterwards they would race back to the office, work some more, then endure a long commute home. This lifestyle often took its toll. Many of them had health issues including high blood pressure, high cholesterol, chronic back pain and obesity. These problems, often stress related, compromised their quality of life, the very life they worked so hard for so long to achieve.

A 2001 study by the Centers for Disease Control and Prevention (CDC) listed life expectancies around the world. Surprisingly, American women finished twenty-fifth with their male counterparts a notch lower at twenty-sixth.

In August 2007 the results of another study were made public. Here, the Census Bureau and the National Center for Health Studies

141

reported that the life expectancy of Americans had dropped to forty-second worldwide.

In both studies, France, Spain and Italy finished near the top, leaving us quite literally in the dust. What was the source of their longevity? Was it diet? While much can be blamed on our consumption of fatty foods, the French have a diet that is high in fat as well. One difference between our nations is the amount of time that most Americans spend in a stressful work environment. In those countries, overtime is rare and many people take a month or more of vacation each summer. That hypothesis is echoed in a study conducted at the Harvard School of Medicine that showed stress to be as likely as a high fat diet to cause a heart attack.

Clearly this is a variable that can be difficult to control. Some jobs require you to work long hours while with others there is pressure to do so. Still, many people are not required to work overtime yet seek out those extra hours. In some jobs it becomes competitive. The most senior people, the ones who probably need a break the most, greedily scoop them up, sometimes doubling their work week in the process. Is this the case with you? If so, then the next time you are fighting tooth and nail for those extra hours stop and ask yourself this question: "If this shortens my life is it really worth it?" It's five o'clock, go home!

Suggested Reading

Chained to the Desk: A Guidebook for Workaholics, Their Partners and Children, and the Clinicians Who Treat Them by Bryan E. Robinson (New York University Press, April 2001)

Want More Info?

Workaholics Anonymous has an interesting site. You can find them at: www.workaholics-anonymous.org.

"Age is a question of mind over matter. If you don't mind, it doesn't matter."
—*Satchel Paige*

Section III:

AFTER WORK: YOUR WORKOUT

*"Those who do not find time for exercise will
have to find time for illness."*
—**The Earl of Darby**

"The only way you hurt the body is when you don't use it."
—**Fitness Guru Jack LaLanne**

The next segment of this book is dedicated to exercise. As a personal trainer, it is a topic with which I'm quite familiar and one that has a lot to do with how well and how long we live. In a survey done in 2006 by the Rudd Center for Food Policy and Obesity at Yale University, a high percentage of those polled said that if they had to choose between taking years off their life and being obese they would choose the former. Of the 4000 plus who responded, 15 percent would be willing to shave a full ten years off their life in order to keep their weight in check. I find this ironic when many of those same people forego regular exercise which would not only fight obesity but *lengthen* their lives. Studies involving people who had lived to age 100 and beyond have consistently shown them to have maintained a stable body weight for most of their adult lives. Those findings take on even greater significance in the wake of a study published in 2006. It showed diabetes, a disease exacerbated by excess body weight, is on the rise and may soon lead to the first decline in average American life expectancy in over 100 years. According to Robert Rizza, president of the American Diabetes Association, "If we as a country stay lean and fit, we likely will prevent up to 90 or 95 percent of diabetes in the years ahead."

Much of the information contained in the following section can be traced back to my studies with the following organizations: the American Council on Exercise (ACE), the National Academy of Sports Medicine (NASM) and the National Strength and Conditioning Association (NSCA). I would like to thank them for providing me with a quality education in regard to health and fitness.

"Truly a flexible back makes a long life."
—Chinese proverb

"Flexibility is achieved through safe stretching techniques,
a little at a time, and always stretch when you are
warm. Also, get some good advice from a teacher."
—Deborah Bull, Ballet Dancer

24 | 5:45 p.m. Will You Stretch?

Flexibility: A joint's ability to move through a full and normal range of motion.

Your workday is done and it's time to hit the gym.

Warm-up

This is a part of many busy people's exercise routine that is often left out, a decision that can prove to be a poor one. For best results and to avoid injury it is important to begin your workout with a five to ten minute warm-up. This raises your body temperature, making muscles more pliable, and redirects your body's blood supply from the heart to the working muscles. A warm-up is especially important for anyone with a history of heart trouble and may need to be extended.

If you live a mile or so from your exercise facility then walking there can be an excellent choice. It will prepare you both physically and mentally for the activity that will follow. Many people will go to the gym and walk contentedly for hours on a treadmill but not if they have to walk two blocks to get there. This is something I have never understood.

If a walk to the gym is not an option, then five to ten minutes of any low intensity exercise will prove sufficient. Good choices include walking on a treadmill, riding an exercise bike or a brisk stroll around the gym. After completing your warm-up, it's time to stretch.

145

Time to Stretch

When designing an exercise program the most controversial component is flexibility. Fitness professionals frequently debate the true value of stretching in improving performance and avoiding injury. Opinions also differ as to which method is the safest and most beneficial. Below are some of the best known styles along with the advantages and disadvantages of each:

Static Stretching: Movements are slow, controlled and work through a full range of motion. This type of stretching is probably the best choice for most people.

Advantage: Combines a high degree of safety with substantial results. That combination has made it the first choice of many in the fitness industry.

Drawback: While it is both safe and effective, results may not match those provided by the alternatives listed below.

Ballistic Stretching: Employs bouncing movements that are rapid and uncontrolled. This can be an effective way to attain the extreme range of motion needed to perform certain sports or activities.

Advantage: Provides strong results for those involved in sports that employ rapid, ballistic movements.

Drawback: In spite of the potential benefits, this type of flexibility training is far riskier than static stretching and is probably not the best choice for people with general fitness goals.

Proprioceptive Neuromuscular Facilitation (PNF): A type of assisted stretching that was developed by medical professionals as a method of rehabilitation. First, the patient contracts a muscle isometrically against resistance applied by the therapist for a period of approximately six seconds. Next, a slow, passive stretch is performed past the previous point of restriction. This type of stretching is now popular in many health clubs and is a tool often used by personal trainers.

Advantage: Increases muscular strength as well as flexibility.

Drawback: PNF is a complex concept. Performing it with someone who is not fully qualified can present risks not worth taking.

Self-Myofascial Release: A system for improving flexibility by applying pressure to spots where fibrous bands of connective tissue, known as fascia, have "bundled up" leaving you with restrictions that can both cause pain and limit range of motion. By realigning the fibers properly, discomfort can be alleviated and flexibility improved. Foam rolls are a common tool used for this technique and are now a fixture in most health clubs.

Advantage: A great way to precisely target impediments to proper functioning.

Drawback: Since fewer people are familiar with this concept than with more traditional methods, proper training is essential. Some equipment is required.

Recommendation

It is the opinion of most fitness professionals that static stretching is the best and safest choice for those whose goal is general fitness. Below are some useful guidelines:

- Hit all muscle groups you plan to train during your workout

- Focus on those muscles that are tight, thereby inhibiting normal range of motion. Don't overstretch those that are already flexible

- Hold all stretches for a minimum of 15-20 seconds unless otherwise indicated

- Don't bounce. This causes the muscle to contract and can lead to both soreness and stiffness

Conclusion

Flexibility training is helpful for those wishing to improve performance and avoid injury. Still, it is important to remember that more is not necessarily better. Athletes, such as martial artists and gymnasts, who need a tremendous range of motion to perform at a competitive level, often suffer from joint instability later in life. This occurs when a reduction in strength training results in a corresponding reduction in their level of muscular development. Once the athlete's muscles atrophy, these muscles can no longer support the joint's once sought after hypermobility. Winning those gold medals may make such risks seem worthwhile, but for the average exerciser with general fitness goals, there is not enough of an upside to compensate for the problems they may eventually face. My recommendation is to stretch regularly but not to take your gains in flexibility farther than safety would dictate.

Stretches

"A picture is worth a thousand words."
—Chinese proverb

The following section contains a program made up of popular and effective stretching exercises. Since describing an exercise cannot compare with showing one, I have included illustrations of both the starting and finishing positions to accompany the written explanations. These are by no means the only valid exercises that are available to you, but they are a great place to start.

BACK

Lie down comfortably on an exercise mat with your legs fully extended and your feet no more than six inches apart.

As you take a deep breath, raise your arms over your head. As you exhale, flex your feet up towards you and flatten your lower back against the mat.

*Hold this stretch for a minimum of 10 seconds.

Starting Position

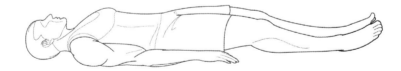

Finishing Position

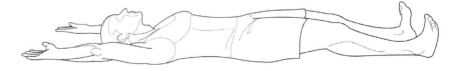

Place your hands behind your knees and take a deep breath. Then as you exhale, raise them towards your chest keeping your head on the mat and your neck and shoulders relaxed.

*Avoid placing your hands over your knees. This puts pressure on them and serves no useful purpose.

*Hold this stretch for a minimum of 15-20 seconds.

Starting Position

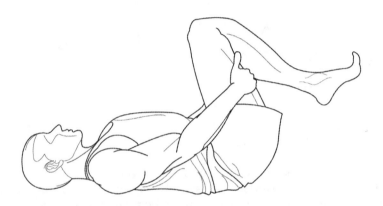

Finishing Position

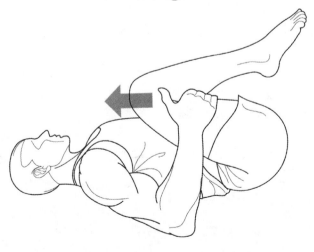

Kneel with your head down and your arms resting comfortably on the mat, palms down. Take a deep breath, then as you exhale, let your body slide backwards without raising your head or arms. Focus on the comfortable stretch you should be feeling throughout your back.

*Hold this stretch for a minimum of 15-20 seconds.

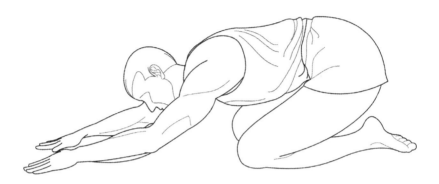

While still in this position, turn your arms over so that your palms face up, then repeat the exercise. This subtle change in position increases involvement of the latissimus dorsi, or lats, the large muscles on the sides of your upper back.

*Hold this stretch for a minimum of 15-20 seconds.

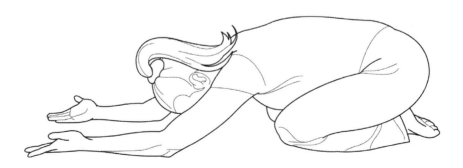

HAMSTRINGS

Sit comfortably on the mat with your left leg extended and the sole of your right foot resting against the inside of your left thigh. Take a deep breath. As you exhale, bend from the waist reaching for your foot with both hands. After a few seconds flex your feet back towards you for a deeper stretch.

*Make sure not to dip your head or round your back.

*Remember not to bounce. Bouncing causes the muscle to contract which can lead to soreness.

*Hold this stretch for a minimum of 15-20 seconds.

Starting Position

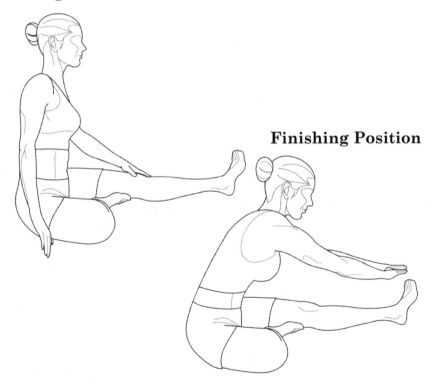

Finishing Position

Switch legs and repeat the exercise.

Extend both legs in front of you with your heels no more than six inches apart. Take a deep breath, then while bending from the waist, reach for your feet with both hands, without dipping your head or rounding your back. After a few seconds, flex your feet back towards you to increase the stretch. This exercise stretches your hamstrings, three muscles running down the back of your legs. Tightness there puts pressure on your lower back, increasing the risk of injury.

*Hold this stretch for a minimum of 15-20 seconds.

Starting Position

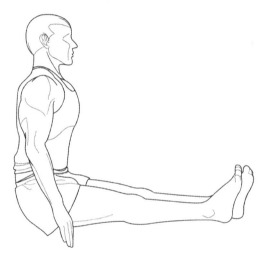

Finishing Position

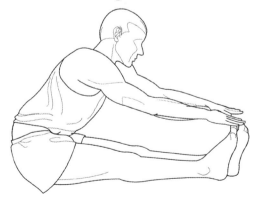

GROIN

Sit on the mat with the soles of your feet together, a comfortable distance from your groin. Next, take a deep breath while cupping your ankles with your hands. Now, as you slowly exhale, use your elbows and forearms to gently push your legs down until you feel a comfortable stretch throughout your groin.

*Always remember not to bounce, as it can lead to soreness in the groin area.

*Hold this stretch for a minimum of 15-20 seconds.

Starting Position

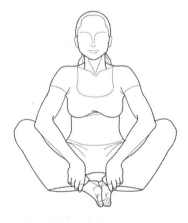

Finishing Position

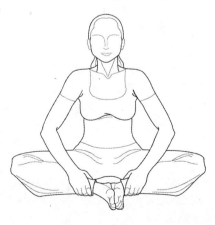

Separate your legs into a V-shape as far as you can comfortably. Take a deep breath, and then as you exhale, lean forward from the waist as far as you can without rounding your back or dipping your head. If you're flexible enough, place your palms on the mat in front of you. If not, do these stretches daily and soon you will be. Hold this stretch for a minimum of 15-20 seconds.

Starting Position

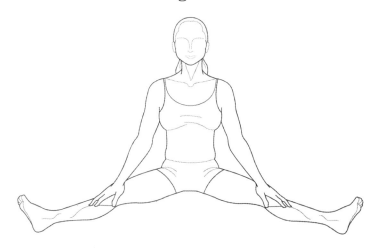

Finishing Position

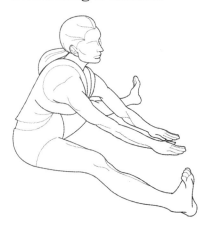

CALVES

Lean against a wall with your front knee bent and your back leg straight. Both feet should be pointing forward. Next, lean forward without allowing your rear heel to rise off the ground.

*Make sure to keep your back leg straight but don't lock your back knee.

*Don't raise your rear heel off the ground.

*Hold this stretch for a minimum of 15-20 seconds.

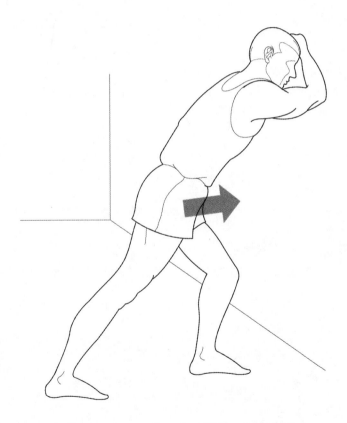

Switch legs. Lean forward. This exercise will stretch your gastrocnemius, a calf muscle that is often tight.

This exercise has the same starting position as the previous one. The difference is that your rear leg will not remain straight but instead will be slightly bent. This will enable you to stretch the soleus, a muscle that lies beneath the gastrocnemius.

*Don't raise your rear heel off the ground.

*Hold this stretch for a minimum of 15-20 seconds.

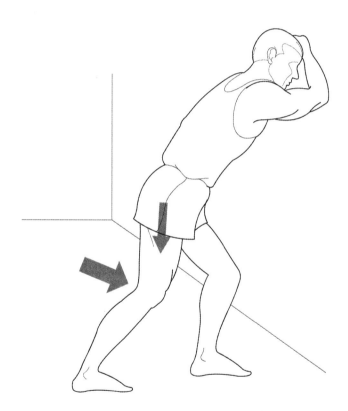

Switch legs and repeat the exercise.

CHEST

Hold onto a pole or the edge of a doorframe with your right hand. Next, begin taking small steps in the opposite direction until you feel a comfortable stretch across your chest. This will effectively stretch your pectoralis major, another muscle that is often short and tight.

*With this stretch it is important not to "fling" yourself violently into the end position since that can do more harm than good. Instead, get there slowly and comfortably.

*Remember to turn from the shoulder not the waist.

*Hold this stretch for a minimum of 15-20 seconds.

Starting Position   Finishing Position

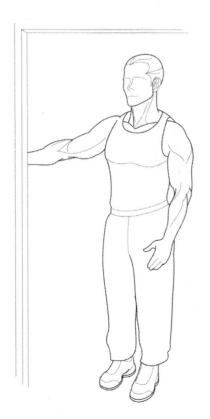 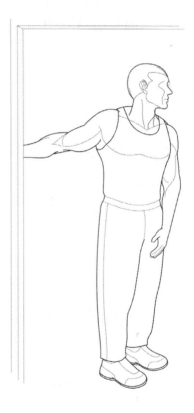

Switch positions and repeat the exercise.

SHOULDERS

Stand comfortably with your feet shoulder width apart and pointed forward. Make sure your hips are in a neutral position, not tilted forward or backward. Your knees should be slightly bent with your chest up, and shoulders back. Next, place the back of your left hand behind your right tricep and use it to bring your right arm across your body. You should feel this in your rear deltoid, a muscle on the back of your shoulder.

*Remember to keep your upper body pointed forward. Turning your upper body with the stretch makes it easier but also less beneficial.

*Hold this stretch for a minimum of 15-20 seconds.

Starting Position   Finishing Position

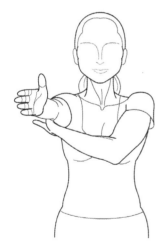 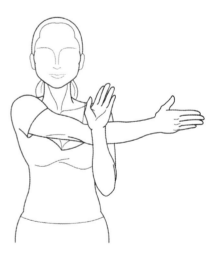

Switch positions and repeat the exercise.

Interlock your fingers in front of you with your palms turned down. Next, raise your arms in front of you, and then if you can, up over your head until your palms face the ceiling.

*Your range of motion should be determined by how far you can go comfortably. Remember not to force it.

*Hold this stretch for a minimum of 15-20 seconds.

Starting Position   **Finishing Position**

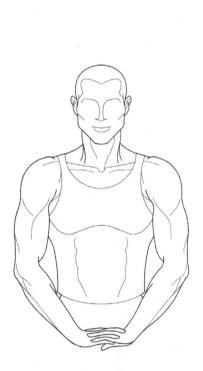 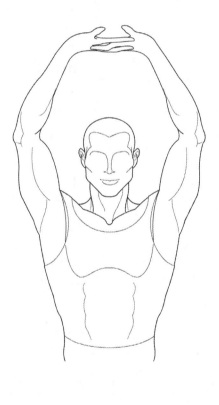

Interlock your fingers behind you. Next, raise your arms as far as you can comfortably.

*Hold this stretch for a minimum of 15-20 seconds.

Starting Position   Finishing Position

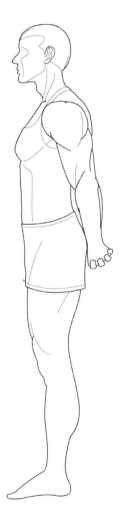
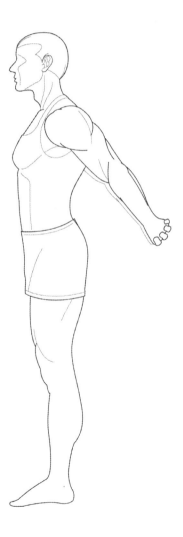

TRICEPS

Stand with your arms stretched overhead. Next, grip your right arm just above the elbow with your left hand and gently pull it behind your head.

*Your right hand should end up on your neck or upper back.

*Remember, in order to get maximum benefit don't turn with the stretch.

*Hold this stretch for a minimum of 15-20 seconds.

Starting Position   Finishing Position

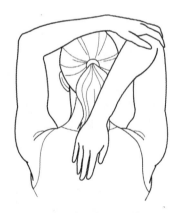
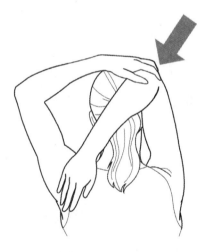

Switch arms and repeat the exercise.

FOREARMS

Get on your hands and knees. Begin turning your fingers to the outside as far as you can comfortably, trying to point them back towards you. Next, very gently lean back until you feel a stretch down the length of your forearms.

*These muscles tend to be especially tight so remember to go easy with this one!

*Hold this stretch for a minimum of 15-20 seconds.

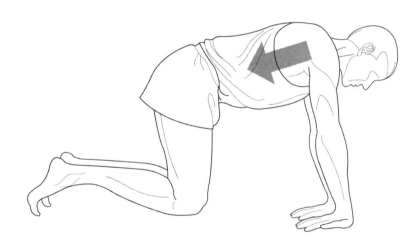

Suggested Reading

Flexibility Training Manual (National Academy of Sports Medicine, 2001)

Science of Flexibility by Michael J. Alter (Human Kinetics, 3rd edition, April 2004)

Stretching: 20th Anniversary by Bob Anderson (Shelter Publications, June 2000)

"Fitness —if it came in a bottle, everybody would have a great body."
—Cher

25 | 5:55 p.m.
Will You Do Any
Strength Training?

When I was a teenager, strength training was limited mostly to athletes and guys who wanted to impress the girls with their bulging biceps. Today, the negative myths that once surrounded this type of exercise have fallen by the wayside and been replaced by reams of scientific evidence showing that regular strength training helps everyone.

A study conducted at Tufts University showed that strength training benefits arthritis sufferers. Resistance training builds bone mass, a boon to those at risk for osteoporosis. As we continue to age, this type of exercise takes on even greater significance, since maintaining muscular strength is crucial to our ability to perform activities of daily living.

A Common Misconception

In the mid-1980s, I was working out in a local health club when a slightly built fellow about 30 years of age asked me to show him how to use an exercise machine. After helping him I inquired as to whether he ever used free weights when he exercised. His response was one I'll always remember. This 130 pound man turned to me and said, "I don't want to look like those guys in the magazines." If only it were that easy! Attaining the level of muscular development this fellow was so afraid of takes a lifetime of commitment, often combined with truckloads of nutritional supplements. A few sets of curls would not make him explode.

I bring this up because many people, particularly women, share his fear. They are afraid that a little weight training will turn them into Mr. Universe. The facts do not bear out their concerns. Women only possess about ten percent of the testosterone that men do. With this significantly lower level of this muscle-building hormone it is extremely difficult for the average woman to bulk up to an unsightly level.

On the positive side, resistance training helps build and preserve bone and muscle mass, a key to fighting both osteoporosis and sarcopenia. This type of exercise is also a great way to reduce your level of body fat, thereby decreasing your risk of diabetes. Weight training makes you feel good by increasing your level of endorphins, hormones that kill pain and create a feeling of euphoria. It helps to prevent arthritis, and lessens the symptoms of menopause. This combination makes resistance training more than worth the effort. So fight your fears and grab a dumbbell!

Strength Training and Osteoporosis

Resistance training builds bone mass, making it a potent weapon in the war against this age-related condition. Bones, like other parts of our anatomy, grow stronger when challenged. Wolf's Law states that bones grow thicker and stronger, or thinner and weaker, in direct proportion to the stress placed on them. As preventive medicine, resistance training helps to slow the loss of minerals that make up your bones. If you already have this condition, it is suggested that you avoid high impact movements. It is also recommended that you consult your physician so he can help you design an appropriate resistance training routine.

Strength Training and Sarcopenia

While osteoporosis is a condition familiar to most of us, sarcopenia, the loss of muscle mass that accompanies the aging process, is rarely discussed. In spite of its relative anonymity, sarcopenia is a condition that can lead to a wide variety of health problems and can eventually prove fatal.

According to the American Council on Exercise (ACE), the average person, who does not engage in regular strength training exercise, loses more than one-half pound of muscle per year after age 25. This muscle tissue is then replaced by approximately one-and-a half pounds of fat. This is an alarming statistic when you consider that the loss of 40 percent of your lean body mass can be life threatening. In addition, the National Strength and Conditioning Association (NSCA) stated in the December 2004 issue of *Strength and Conditioning Journal*, that between their thirties and eighties, this condition results on average in a 15 percent decrease in resting metabolic rate. This results in a corresponding reduction in calorie expenditure of about 250 per day.

While many factors account for these alarming statistics, much of the damage can be traced to a single source, that most people are less active than they should be. Regular exercise has been shown to preserve lean body mass, thus mitigating the harmful effects of this condition, as well as improving the ability of the elderly to perform activities of daily living.

Strength Training and Weight Loss

Weight loss is the primary reason why many people exercise. Our society is obsessed with appearance and it's no secret that thin is in. People want to be lean and they want to lose weight but are they really one and the same? The answer may well surprise you.

The first thing to come to grips with is that it is body fat, not weight, that is unsightly. If you were to build ten pounds of muscle and lose ten pounds of fat your weight would be the same but you would look like a very different person. If you are 50 pounds overweight it is unlikely that you will be able to (or in many cases want to) gain 50 pounds of muscle. However, over time, 10 pounds of muscle can help rid you of that 50 pound spare tire. Here's how:

A pound of muscle burns about 50 calories a day in tiny fat burning engines called mitochondria. Those calories are burned while sitting, sleeping or reading a newspaper. As a result, building ten pounds of muscle, evenly distributed throughout your body will create a 500 calorie a day deficit that you don't have at present. This assumes that your calorie intake remains stable. Since a pound of fat has 3500 calories, this scenario should enable you to lose about one pound per week without changing your diet. Keep in mind that combining the program listed above with a 500 calorie a day *reduction* will double your progress, enabling you to lose two pounds a week instead of one.

Strength Training and Diabetes

Over 18 million Americans have diabetes with more than five million yet to be diagnosed. The diabetic's body is either unable to secrete or to properly utilize insulin, a hormone produced by the pancreas. If left untreated, both forms of the disease, type I and type II, allow blood sugar to rise to levels that are dangerous and potentially life threatening. Physical activity increases your body's sensitivity to insulin. This fact makes regular exercise an excellent way to reduce the type II diabetic's dependence on insulin injections as well as lessen the potentially devastating effects of the disease. Since over 90 percent of all diabetics are type II, time spent in the weight room is a cheap, effective way to avoid falling prey to an illness that threatens to become an epidemic.

Strength Training and Depression

Recent studies have found that over 35 million Americans suffer from serious depression at some point in their lives. Fortunately, drugs and expensive psychotherapy are not the only solutions. It has been shown that 30 minutes of exercise three to five times a week can be effective in reducing symptoms in many of those with clinical depression. This can be attributed in part to increased levels of endorphins and certain neurotransmitters which are known to be mood enhancing. Exercise also results in an elevation in body temperature which can prove soothing.

Strength Training and Arthritis

Osteoarthritis, the most common form of this disease, affects 80 percent of Americans 65 and older. For people suffering from arthritis, strengthening the muscles that surround the affected joints is critical. As we have seen, exercise helps control your weight. This is important for arthritis sufferers since additional weight puts an even greater strain on already damaged joints.

Strength Training and Menopause

Menopause is defined by the World Health Organization as, "Permanent cessation of menstruation resulting in the loss of ovarian follicular activity." It generally occurs around age fifty and brings with it a number of unwelcome side effects.

Hot flashes are menopause's most common symptom. While hormone replacement therapy can combat them effectively, the health risks associated with long term use are substantial. Regular exercise has been shown to provide similar benefits.

This time in a woman's life is often accompanied by another unwelcome surprise, weight gain. This is particularly common around the abdominal area as decreased estrogen levels result in a redistribution of body fat. The good news is that the problem can be slowed or even reversed by engaging in regular exercise.

Breathing

An important aspect of strength training that is often neglected is proper breathing. While there are several theories as to how to breathe while exercising, a good rule of thumb is to exhale on exertion, while simultaneously drawing your navel back towards your spine. Doing so will give you greater support, thereby decreasing the risk of injury. Avoid holding your breath since doing so can increase your blood pressure.

Posture/Balance

When I was in my late teens I began attending a Tae Kwon Do school that was popular in the neighborhood. This particular establishment taught you many techniques quickly, and before long I was punching and kicking to my heart's content. I decided to show some of what I had learned to a friend who was well versed in the martial arts. He looked at me, frowned and said, "They're teaching you how to fight and they haven't even taught you how to stand."

When exercising, as with any form of movement, maintaining proper balance and body positioning is key. We all love to talk about the importance of good "form", a common buzzword in the fitness industry. But good form is more than not jerking the weights up and down. It also refers to how you position yourself. Think of your body the way you would a building. Would you load tons of heavy furniture into the upper floors if you knew its foundation was weak? Don't do that to your body unless you want this irreplaceable structure to collapse.

Standing
When exercising in a standing position, proper alignment is crucial. Some key points to keep in mind:

- Feet shoulder width apart

- Knees flexible (not locked)

- Head up

- Shoulders back

Seated
When performing an exercise in a seated position, proper form is also critical. The pressure placed on your lower back is approximately 30 percent greater than it would be were you to do the same exercise in a standing position. Some key points to keep in mind:

- Don't allow your back to cave-in

- For exercises like lateral raises, curls or shoulder presses, keep your feet flat on the floor and pointed straight ahead

- Head up

- Shoulders back

Make sure to observe yourself in a mirror frequently and on film when possible, in order to assure that your form does not deteriorate.

Designing a Program

The first decision you need to make when designing your strength training program is whether to work your entire body in one day (full body workout) or divide it into two separate components (split routine). Those who split up their workout typically train four days a week, alternating between two different workouts. An example would be to work chest, back, legs and abdominals Monday and Thursday and shoulders, triceps and biceps Tuesday and Friday. Another option is to train six days a week with legs being worked separately twice a week.

Strength Training Variables

When beginning an exercise program, an untrained person will quickly make dramatic gains, particularly in strength. This can be largely attributed to the huge window of adaptation available to those attempting activities to which they are unaccustomed. After a while, their gains will slow to a crawl as the body adapts to the challenges to which it has been subjected. This phenomenon is often referred to as "plateauing". If you are satisfied with the gains you have made you can continue the same exercise program (maintenance). There are, however, numerous variables that you can manipulate should you wish to further challenge your body, allowing for additional gains. Those variables include:

Choice of exercise: This decision should be based on several factors including your fitness goals and physical limitations. There are many exercises that can be used to develop any muscle or group of muscles. Remember to vary them periodically so that your body does not become accustomed to any one routine. A description of many popular and effective strength training exercises are included at the end of this chapter along with illustrations to help you better visualize them.

Order of exercise: There are certain general rules of thumb, such as targeting larger body parts early in your workout. Still, most people don't realize how much additional benefit is available to them just by shifting the order of the exercises that make up their routine. If you do a full body workout, periodically change the order of the body parts you'll be training. Have you started your workout with legs for the past ten years? Why not try starting with chest?

If you do a split routine, then you can also benefit by changing the order of the exercises within each body part. For a change of pace, do reverse curls before curls. If you've been doing flat bench press before incline bench press try reversing the order. Also consider changing which body parts you do together. If you normally do chest and back on the same day, consider switching to chest with biceps.

Number of reps: A rep, short for repetition, refers to performing a given movement or combination of movements once. Examples would be one squat or bicep curl. When it comes to strength training, a common theory is that doing fewer reps with more weight is better for bulking up and gaining strength, while doing more reps with lighter resistance is superior for building endurance and improving muscular definition. Everything we have learned seems to support that belief. Those with a variety of health concerns including obesity, hypertension and heart disease should stick to higher rep totals and lighter resistance for safety reasons. Higher reps are also a good choice for new exercisers so that they can ingrain the desired movement patterns on their nervous system. In general "high" rep totals refer to between 15 and 20 per set. Totals higher than that, while they may help build stamina, will be relatively ineffective in building muscle mass.

Number of sets: A set refers to a series of reps performed in succession before resting. How many times you do an exercise has an obvious impact on the results you can expect. Many people do too many sets of exercises that they consider important. Performing six or more sets of the same exact movement the same exact way is overkill for the average person with typical fitness goals. Doing so can leave you too little time for other important parts of your workout. It can also lead to overtraining, a syndrome that can slow your progress dramatically. When beginning an exercise routine, two to three sets per exercise is ideal. As you progress, you may choose to perform four sets of exercises that you enjoy or consider particularly important. In recent years an argument has been made for doing only one set per exercise. However, the majority of experts agree that one set is not sufficient to achieve the results most people are looking for.

Movement speed: Every repetition has three components the concentric, eccentric and isometric. By manipulating the duration of each, the results you achieve during your workouts can be greatly enhanced. This is a variable that in spite of its importance is too often ignored. The three components are:

Concentric: During this phase, also known as the positive, the resistance is overcome and the muscle shortens. Examples include extending your arms into the up position while performing a bench press or lowering the bar towards your chest during a lat pull-down.

Eccentric: This phase is also called the negative. Here the muscle is overcome by the resistance and lengthens back to its original length. You'll often see people lowering the weight as fast as gravity will allow. This completely disregards the tremendous potential that eccentric training has to offer. Examples of an eccentric muscle action are lowering the bar towards your legs after performing a bicep curl or allowing your upper body to move back towards the ground after doing a crunch.

Isometric: A Greek word meaning same length. During an Isometric muscle action there is resistance, but no change in the length of the muscle. This is undoubtedly the most neglected component of most people's workout, in spite of its great muscle building potential. Examples include pausing at the top of a bench press for a second or two before lowering the weight or holding your arm at a 90 degree angle for a few seconds while performing a bicep curl.

Time between sets: Varying the time that you rest between sets can drastically alter their level of difficulty. People going for muscular endurance frequently take thirty seconds or less while those training for maximal strength often wait as long as three to five minutes. Even if your goal is not about to change, making use of this variable will allow those who have reached a plateau to make additional gains.

A word of caution: People often allow factors unrelated to their exercise prescription to adversely affect this variable. Those just beginning their workout frequently rest longer than their plan calls for while those nearing the end rush so they can finish their routine and head home. Some individuals turn the gym into a social experience and can easily talk through the equivalent of two or three sets without even realizing it. In order to get the maximum benefit from your workout make sure that the time you take between sets is that which you have planned.

More Tools for Your Toolbox

Supersets: Do one exercise to failure, then after putting down the weights, immediately grab the appropriate weights and do a different exercise that involves an opposing muscle group. Examples would be doing tricep extensions followed immediately by bicep curls or leg extensions (quads) followed by leg curls (hamstrings).

Compound sets: This concept is similar to the superset, except that it employs the same rather than two opposing muscle groups. Examples include following a set of dumbbell bench press with push-ups (both chest exercises) or doing front raises for your front deltoids, followed immediately by lateral raises to emphasize your middle deltoids.

Drop sets: Start with one level of resistance then once you have reached the number of repetitions that you can do while maintaining proper form, reduce the resistance so that you can do additional reps. An example would be doing shoulder presses with 30 pound dumbbells then putting them down and immediately picking up 15 pound dumbbells and continuing the set.

Home Fitness Equipment

Some people have neither the time nor the desire to go to a gym, but still want to stay in shape. For them, home fitness equipment can be an ideal solution. While there are more products on the market than you can count, the four listed below are a particularly good value, taking into account space required, effectiveness and versatility.

Bowflex: Perhaps the most versatile piece of home fitness equipment available. Offers you a high intensity workout using up to 310 pounds of resistance then folds up and fits in the closet. The Bowflex enables you to effectively work your entire body while the instability of the bows forces your core muscles to kick in and stabilize each movement. Most models cost over $1000 but each is many machines in one. Resistance can be increased to 410 pounds by purchasing 2 additional power rods. For more info visit their website at: www.bowflex.com.

Power Blocks: Power Blocks are ideal for free-weight lovers who lack the space that multiple sets of dumbbells require. By simply pulling a pin these adjustable 21 pound dumbbells can be converted in three pound increments all the way down to three pounds. Other models are also available, in weights ranging up to 130 pounds per dumbbell. For more information visit their website at: www.powerblock.com.

Tubing: The most inexpensive fitness equipment available. Effective, yet each piece of tubing takes up less space than a jump rope. These bands of rubber can be used to simulate virtually any free weight exercise. Resistance varies according to the thickness of each band and they are color coded to avoid any possible confusion.

AbRoller: When working your abdominal muscles, this popular invention helps limit unwanted hip rotation. This focuses your efforts

171

on your abs rather than just tiring out your neck and arms. Most models include a padded neck support.

Core Training: You're Only as Strong as Your Weakest Link

Core training is a popular phrase in the fitness industry. It refers to strengthening your body's deep postural muscles, those from which all movement emanates. A key to effectively training your core is to exercise in an unstable environment. This forces your stabilizer muscles to "kick in" and control the movement. Training in this way gives you a solid foundation to work from and avoids any weak links in your kinetic chain. Several popular and effective core training exercises are listed in the section at the end of this chapter.

Core Training Equipment

Stability Ball: These inflatable balls, which come in a variety of sizes, are now standard equipment in nearly every gym. By incorporating them into a wide range of exercises including squats, push-ups and crunches, stabilizer muscles, often neglected in traditional workouts, can be brought into play.

BOSU: Short for Both Sides Up, this versatile domed device is an effective way to improve balance, which tends to deteriorate as we age. By exercising on an unstable surface like the BOSU, balance cannot only be maintained, but improved. Exercises can be performed on the flat side or on the inflatable rubber dome, either with or without movement. Closing one's eyes while balancing on the dome can further increase the challenge.

Foam Roll: These cylinders made of hard foam come in a variety of lengths. They are used to improve balance and strengthen your stabilizer muscles. Doing push-ups on them is a favorite exercise of mine. Controlling the cylinder's natural tendency to roll is a challenge that adds a new dimension to a classic exercise. Standing on them is another option. They are also used as a tool for self-myofascial release, discussed previously in our section on stretching.

To purchase core training or other fitness equipment the websites below are good choices:

www.power-systems.com

www.performbetter.com

www.spriproducts.com

Integration versus Isolation

There is a movement in the fitness world away from exercises such as leg extensions and leg curls that attempt to isolate specific muscles or muscle groups. Instead, fitness experts now favor multi-joint exercises like squats, leg presses, lunges and deadlifts. During these exercises there is coordinated movement at several joints simultaneously. It is important to keep in mind that only during multiple joint movements such as these should motion occur at more than one joint, and then only that movement which is considered beneficial. One of the biggest mistakes made in many gyms is to "cheat" by using unwanted movement at joints other than those involved in the exercise in order to get the weights to move. Examples would be rocking your body back and forth during a cable row or movement at the shoulder during a bicep curl. While this may allow you to lift heavier weights, you will be fooling yourself as well as risking injury.

Working Around or Through Injuries

In the late seventies a young man began a weight-training program. Early in one of his exhaustive workouts he injured his lower back. Not wanting to miss a single rep, he finished the entire two-hour routine. For nearly a week afterward he was barely able to get out of bed.

In the mid-eighties I knew a fellow who broke his arm. At a point before it had fully healed he decided he could no longer stand to miss any part of his weight training regimen. He then had a hook attached to the cast so he could do curls.

In the fall of 2005 I met a guy in the gym who was complaining of a serious shoulder problem. He refused to stop doing squats even though the bar resting on his shoulder caused him tremendous pain. He was finally going to an orthopedist because he could no longer raise his arm above 90 degrees.

All the above stories are true and involved people I knew personally. Unfortunately, the foolish young man in anecdote number one was me. There is a strong motivation for individuals dedicated to fitness to fight their way through the pain of an injury rather than lose what they have worked so hard to gain. While there are certainly times when you can "work around" an injury, meaning do exercises that don't directly aggravate it, remember to be cautious. The last thing you want is to miss an extended period of time or worse still, cause yourself a life changing injury just to avoid missing a few weeks in the weight room.

Remember the old saying, "Muscle has memory"? You will get it back much quicker than you developed it the first time around, but not if a serious injury leaves you unable to function normally.

That being said, there are also times when the total lack of exercise, in a body that is used to regular exercise, can be detrimental both physically and mentally. So how does one handle such a paradox? Listen to both your doctor and your body. With many injuries it will be possible to remain active to some degree. For example, someone with an arm injury can still walk and someone with a leg injury can work on a seated chest press machine.

Steroids

With all that is known about the dangers of steroid use, it amazes me that it's still the problem that it is. The consequences of steroid abuse are frightening. They include kidney and liver damage, hair loss, mood swings, changes in sexual characteristics and an increased risk of developing cancer. In addition, the results of a Yale University study, released in 2006, showed that steroid abuse can result in a significant loss of brain cells. If you are a competitive athlete who is abusing steroids, be aware that you're putting your life on the line in order to win by cheating. If not, then you are paying an awfully high price to be the best looking guy at the water cooler.

Weight Belts

One of the questions I'm frequently asked is, "Should I wear a weight belt?" You have all seen them and when I first started lifting weights everyone wore them. That is one of the reasons why so many people had bad backs. It is not that the belt fails to provide support. On the contrary, the support it provides is *too* effective. By gaining this "edge" artificially, a muscle in the body called the transverse abdominus no longer needs to supply that support naturally. As a result, once you lift something without your belt the transverse is no longer functioning at the level necessary to properly do its job. If you have never worn a belt before, have no back issues, and plan on using good form, it is probably best not to wear one except during very heavy lifts. If, on the other hand, you have worn a belt until now or have a back injury, don't just toss your belt aside. If you do so, you will be setting yourself up for injury. At this point, you will need to be weaned off the belt gradually and under professional supervision.

Don't Be Fooled by Appearances

A number of years ago, I was at the gym while this well-developed guy was trying to impress a young woman by showing her how to workout. He asked me to validate a point he had just made that was not only a bad idea, but a dangerous one. Since I could not do so in good conscience, I declined. The next time he saw me, I was scolded for contradicting him. He informed me that although the exercise he was showing her might damage her shoulder, most competitive power lifters have shoulder problems. I looked at him quizzically and asked if he'd ever considered the possibility that this 20 year old girl might not want to be a competitive power lifter. From the expression on his face, it was clear that he hadn't.

You're at the gym and you see someone with the look you crave doing an exercise with which you are not familiar. You want to know what he does to get those biceps to bulge or that six pack to look so ripped. Before you decide to make this hunk your guru, be aware that his Adonis-like physique might have less to do with his routine and more to do with his family tree. Fitness experts often say that some guys are big because they were smart enough to pick the right parents. Genetics play a major role in the results we achieve and while everyone can benefit from regular exercise, it does not mean that if you follow this fellow's advice you will end up looking like him. Instead, you might end up with an injury from forces that his physique has so far been able to withstand.

Where to Go for Answers

Personal Trainers

It's standard practice in many gyms for management to ask trainers to do orientations for new members, then pitch a series of personal training sessions to them. While some trainers come on a bit strong, they can also be a great source of information that can help you get the most for your time and money. If after your orientation you feel competent to train yourself, great. If not, and you are looking for fitness advice (aside from the information in this book, of course), then a personal trainer can be a good choice. Make sure, however, that the trainer you choose is qualified. Personal training is a highly unregulated industry and many of the available certifications aren't worth the paper on which they're printed. To make the search a little easier, I'm listing four certifications that, like a college degree in exercise physiology, are a good sign that the individual is competent. While these are by no means the only reputable credentials available they are among the most respected:

* The American College of Sports Medicine (ACSM)

* The American Council on Exercise (ACE)

- The National Academy of Sports Medicine (NASM)

- The National Strength and Conditioning Association (NSCA)

Become Certified

If you are truly committed to learning the ins and outs of all facets of exercise science, then getting certified is an excellent idea. All the certifying bodies mentioned in the previous section are fine choices and preparing for their examinations will provide you with a wealth of knowledge that will prove invaluable in planning and executing a routine that will help you reach your goals.

Journals

Journals published by the certifying bodies listed above are a great resource. They offer the reader cutting edge information on the latest fitness trends gleaned from studies done by some of the top researchers in the field.

They include:

- *ACE Fitness Matters* (ACE)

- *ACSM's Health & Fitness Journal* (ACSM)

- *IDEA Fitness Journal* (IDEA)

- *The Journal of Strength And Conditioning Research* (NSCA)

- *Strength and Conditioning Journal* (NSCA)

To receive the NSCA publications one does not need to become a certified trainer. They can merely join the NSCA as a professional member and the journals will be mailed to you on a regular basis. You can purchase a subscription to *ACE Fitness Matters*, a bi-monthly publication, for $19.95 per year. *IDEA Fitness Journal* is published ten times a year and is mailed to all IDEA members. *ACSM's Health & Fitness Journal* is published bi-monthly.

The Web

When it comes to fitness there are many websites that are highly informative. Some of those that offer quality fitness information include:

ACSM: www.acsm.org

ACE: www.acefitness.org

NSCA: www.nsca-lift.org

NASM: www.nasm.org

IDEA: www.ideafit.com

WebMD: www.webmd.com

Recommendation

While many choices exist in designing your strength training routine, a good starting point for new exercisers is to do a full body workout three times a week. Remember not to do the same routine two days in a row, so Monday, Wednesday, Friday or Tuesday, Thursday, Saturday are ideal. Doing one exercise for each body part is recommended with additional exercises added for muscle groups that you choose to emphasize. Do two to three sets per exercise with rest periods of approximately one minute. Start with 15-20 repetitions so that you can safely build endurance while your body memorizes the correct movement patterns. You can then increase the resistance and reduce the reps if your goal is to build a substantial amount of muscle mass. The movement speed that best suits most people's goals is a four second positive and a two second negative with a one to two second isometric pause.

Those who exercise regularly should feel free to refer back to the variables listed above. Do so whenever you feel bored with your routine or reach a plateau. This will keep the routine fresh, thereby improving focus as well as allowing for additional progress to be made.

Four Exercises I *Don't* Recommend

Before we discuss the exercises that can help you safely achieve your goals, let's examine those that are best left out of your routine. They are either an inefficient use of your time or present a risk of injury that outweighs the benefits they provide. The first three are exercises I did regularly before I learned how damaging they could be. Since I stopped doing them over a decade ago my chronic shoulder problems have improved dramatically.

Behind-the-Neck Press: Many people who choose this exercise are under the misconception that it targets their rear deltoids, the portion of the muscle located on the back of their shoulders. Others do it just because it is being done by the big guy next to them. In reality, the motion this exercise involves is shoulder flexion which works the front deltoid just as it would if they used dumbbells parallel to the head or did a front press. The primary difference when the bar is held behind the neck is the added stress placed on the shoulder joint. There is no additional benefit.

Behind-the-Neck Pull-Down: A gym standard done by men and women of all ages. This exercise has the same drawback as the behind the neck press in that tremendous stress is placed on the shoulder joint with no advantage over pulling the bar down in front of you and bringing it to your upper chest. Since the rotator cuff, which works to stabilize your shoulder joint, tends to breakdown as we age, this exercise is especially risky for seniors.

Upright Row: This exercise, done to develop the upper trapezius, has been popular for as long as I can remember. While it can be effective, the stress that it places on the shoulder joint is a major consideration, particularly for those with shoulder problems. A better option for safe, effective development of the upper traps is shrugs. They will be discussed in detail later in this chapter.

Tricep Kickback (Using a Dumbbell): While this exercise is not necessarily dangerous it *is* ineffective. For an exercise to be worth your time and effort, the resistance and the motion must be moving in opposing directions. In this case, as you throw your arm backward the resistance, namely gravity, is pulling downward. To make a dumbbell kickback effective, the exerciser must lean not just forward but downward, placing their back in a position of vulnerability. A better option is some sort of cable apparatus where gravity is redirected by the machine.

Some Strength Training Dos and Don'ts:

Do Abs Last: The rest of your body counts on your abdominal muscles for support. Once you fatigue your abs by working them effectively they will be less able to offer that support. As a result, abdominal work is best done at the end of your strength training routine.

Don't Lift Right After Eating: After you eat your body draws blood away from your muscles and into the digestive tract in order to aid in the digestive process. Strength training draws that same blood away from the body's core and into the working muscles. Because of this potential conflict, it is advisable to wait a minimum of one hour after eating before beginning to exercise.

Do Eat No More than 3-4 Hours Before Lifting: By taking in some nourishment, especially from sources high in complex carbohydrates, you will assure that your muscle's glycogen stores are adequate. This will enable you to perform up to your potential.

Don't Cheat: In gym circles, cheating refers to changing the way that you do an exercise in order to lift more weight than you could have had the exercise been performed properly. This can be done through the use of momentum, such as swinging your body while doing a bicep curl or by bouncing the bar off your chest while performing a bench press. It also refers to employing muscles other than those that are normally involved in the exercise. An example would be movement at the shoulder when performing a bicep curl or arching your back while performing a shoulder press. Cheating is dangerous and should be avoided.

Exercises

Following are starting and finishing positions for a number of valid strength-training exercises, along with tips on how to perform them correctly. While no one exercise is right for everyone, this information should get you headed in the right direction. The body will be broken up into upper, middle and lower segments with an exercise and one or two alternate exercises listed for each body part.

Upper Body

Chest
Chest Press (Dumbbells)

While a straight bar is often used for this exercise, dumbbells are more effective for general fitness goals. From the starting position shown, take a deep breath then as you exhale, raise the dumbbells while at the same time angling them towards each other until the inner edges nearly touch. Next, slowly lower the weights down and out to the side until your elbows are even with or slightly lower than your upper body.

*Remember never to raise your back up off the bench. Arching your back in order to help lift the weights is harmful to your back and decreases the exercise's effectiveness.

*Don't jerk the weight up at the bottom of the movement.

*Never lock your elbows.

*Bring the weights down slowly and under control.

*Don't get sloppy with the form or the count.

Starting Position   **Finishing Position**

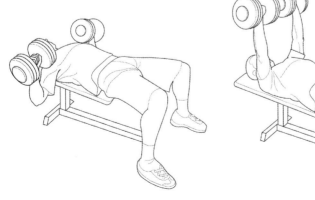

Incline Chest Press (Dumbbells)

The purpose of this exercise is to focus on the upper fibers of your pectorals. For every degree that you raise the bench, more of your pecs' lower fibers are taken out of the exercise, forcing the upper ones to work harder. While the angle you set can vary, 15-20 percent is a good rule of thumb.

The form here is similar to that used for flat bench.

Starting Position

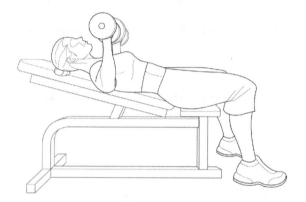

Finishing Position

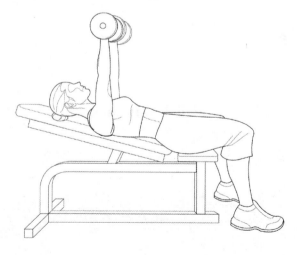

Push-Ups (Body Weight)

Assume the starting position shown below. Next, inhale as you lower your body slowly and under control, until your chest is just off the ground (mid-position). Next as you exhale, draw your navel back towards your spine and return to the starting position.

*Hands shoulder width apart.

*Thumbs aligned with nipple line.

*Knees hip width apart.

*Your body should form a straight line throughout the movement.

*Remember Not to lock your elbows and Not to lead with your hips.

Starting/Finishing Position

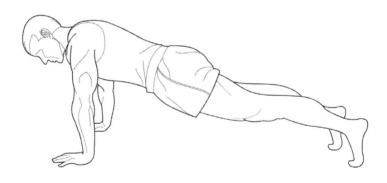

Mid-Position

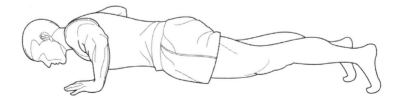

Back

Lat Pull-Downs (Cables)

Grasp the bar with your hands a little more than shoulder width apart. Take a deep breath then as you exhale, lower the bar to your upper chest slowly and under control.

*Initiate this movement by depressing your scapula (lowering your shoulder blades). The tendency with this exercise is to let your biceps do much of the work. Since your lats are the focus, use the depression of your scapula to get the bar moving.

*Avoid momentum (don't jerk the bar to get it moving).

*Don't bring the bar lower than chest level. Doing so requires your shoulders to internally rotate which is not generally the goal of this exercise.

*Slightly vary the grip width periodically.

Starting Position   Finishing Position

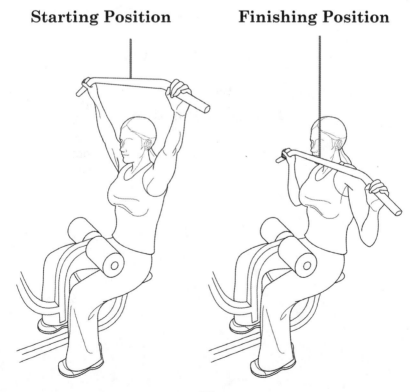

Rows (Cables)

Grasp the bar with a shoulder width grip. Take a deep breath then as you exhale, bring the bar to your chest.

*It is crucial to maintain your spinal position throughout the exercise.

*No rocking back and forth as is often done. That type of "kick start" might help move the weight, but only through momentum, and can be damaging to your spine.

Starting Position

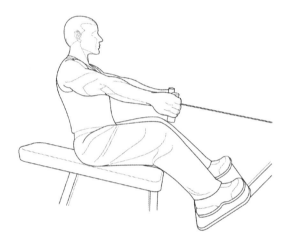

Finishing Position

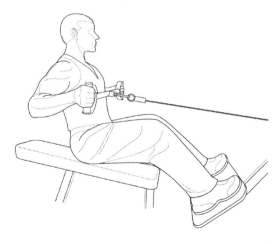

Erector Spinae (Lower Back Muscles)

Lower Back Extensions

Lie on your stomach with your arms at your sides, the backs of your hands facing down.

Take a deep breath then as you exhale, use your lower back muscles to raise your upper body to a comfortable point, then hold that position for 3 - 5 seconds.

*Keep your upper body in a straight line as you raise yourself. Only go as high as you can comfortably, don't force it.

*Remember not to use your neck muscles to "jump start" the movement.

*If a 3 second pause is too difficult start with 1 and work your way up.

*Do 4 sets of 10 with a 1-minute rest period, increasing to 15 reps as you get stronger.

Starting Position

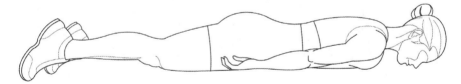

Finishing Position

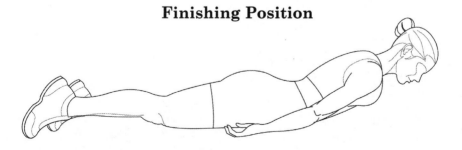

Shoulders

Shoulder Press (Dumbbells)

Start by holding two dumbbells parallel to your neck as shown. Take a deep breath, then as you exhale, begin to raise them straight up and start moving them closer together until at the top of the movement the edges nearly touch. As you inhale begin your return to starting position.

*Exactly how close the edges of the weights come to each other depends on the construction and flexibility of your shoulder joint. Don't force it.

*Don't let your back cave in as you raise the weights.

*Don't jerk the weights up.

*Don't use your legs to "kick start" the movement. This is often done by people using weight far too heavy for the exercise.

Starting Position	**Finishing Position**
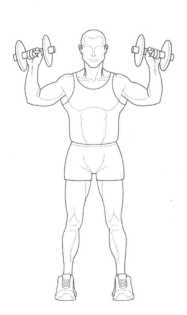	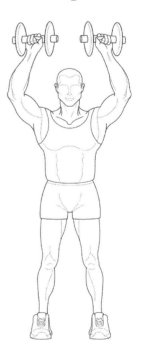

Lateral Raises (Dumbbells)

This exercise focuses on the middle portion of your deltoids.

*Slightly elevate and retract your scapula (shoulder blades).

*Raise the weights no higher than the bottom of your ears. Only lower them to just below waist level.

*Don't swing your upper body. Many people do this in order to lift weight heavier than they could when doing the exercise properly. Remember this is not a power exercise.

*Don't use your legs.

Starting Position   Finishing Position

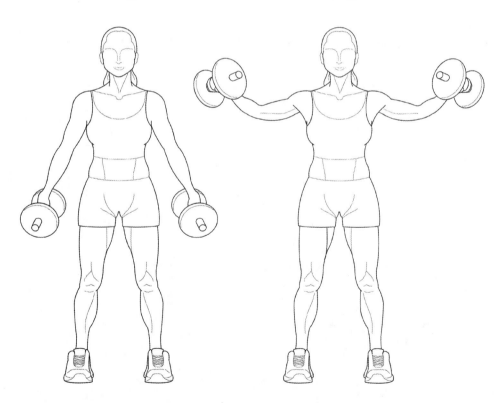

Shrugs (Dumbbells)

This exercise focuses on the upper trapezius (traps), a muscle located on the upper part of your shoulders.

Stand with your feet shoulder width apart. Take a deep breath, then as you exhale, raise your traps towards the back of your head, not your ears.

*Pause briefly before lowering the weights.

*The weight should be raised straight up, not rotated in a circular pattern as is often done. Rotations can damage the shoulder joint while offering no additional benefit.

*Always remember to bring the weight up towards your head not your head down towards the weight. To check this, watch your chin and make sure it doesn't dip as the weights elevate.

<table>
<tr><td>

Starting Position

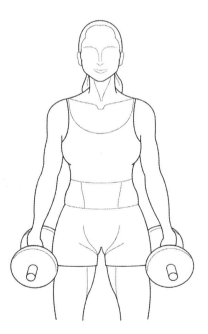

</td><td>

Finishing Position

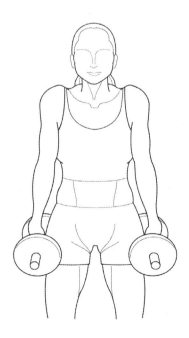

</td></tr>
</table>

Triceps

Tricep Extensions (Dumbbells)

Hold two dumbbells parallel, about six inches from either side of your head. Take a deep breath, then as you exhale, draw your navel back towards your spine for support and extend your elbows until your arms are nearly straight.

*Keep your wrists straight (don't flex them during the exercise).

*As you extend your elbows, no motion should occur at the shoulder.

*Don't allow your elbows to travel outward as they extend.

*Don't lock your elbows at the top of the movement.

Starting Position

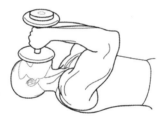

Finishing Position

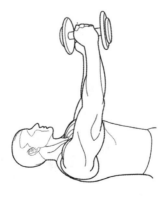

Push-Downs (Cables)

Take a deep breath, then as you exhale, draw your navel back towards your spine and begin to extend your elbows.

*As you push the bar down, your elbows will have a tendency to point out to the side, rather than straight back. Limit this as much as possible. Using a rope rather than the standard V-shaped attachment will help.

*During the negative phase, only allow the weight rise to a height about level with your diaphragm.

*Avoid using movement at the wrist or shoulder.

Starting Position   Finishing Position

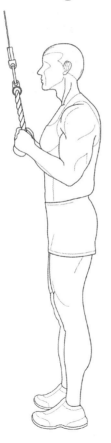 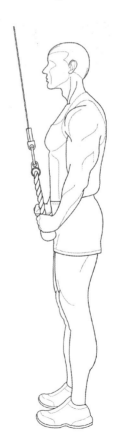

Elbow Flexors (Biceps, etc.)

Bicep Curl (Straight Bar)

Grip the bar with your palms up, about shoulder width apart. Your arms should be almost fully extended, but your elbows should not be locked. Take a deep breath, then as you exhale, raise the bar as high as you can without causing any movement at the shoulder.

*Vary your grip width periodically.

*Can also be done with dumbbells.

*Avoid using momentum (don't swing your upper body).

Starting Position   Finishing Position

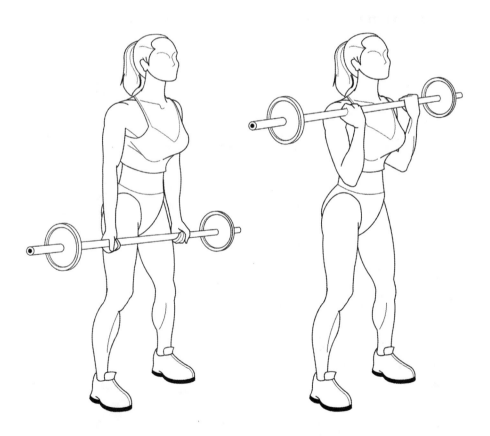

Reverse Curls (Straight Bar)

This exercise emphasizes the bracialis, a muscle that lies beneath your bicep and aids in elbow flexion.

Grip the bar with your palms facing your legs, about shoulder width apart. Take a deep breath then as you exhale, raise the bar until the backs of your hands face your shoulders.

*No movement should occur at the shoulder.

*Vary your grip width periodically.

*Can also be done with dumbbells.

*Avoid using momentum (don't swing your upper body).

Starting Position   Finishing Position

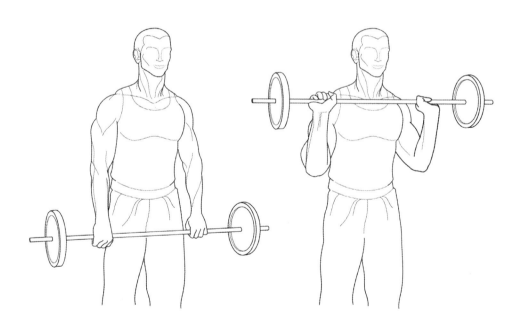

Hammer Curls (Dumbbells)

Start with your arms at your sides and your hands holding dumbbells, just outside of your thighs. Take a deep breath, then as you exhale, raise your forearms until they form a 90 percent angle with your upper arms and the dumbbells are pointed straight ahead. Pause, and slowly return to the starting position.

*All movement occurs at the elbows; your shoulders should remain stable.

*Avoid using momentum.

Starting Position   ## Finishing Position

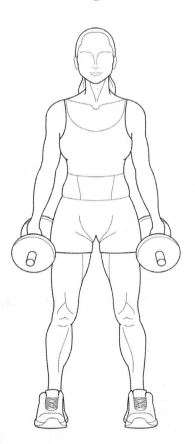
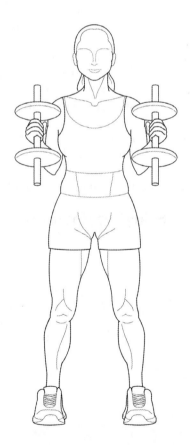

Mid-Body

Abdominals

One of the keys to effectively developing your abdominal muscles is to minimize hip rotation. This is the reason why traditional sit ups have long since been replaced by crunches.

The Crunch

Lie down on the mat with your knees bent and your feet flat on the floor.

Take a deep breath then as you exhale, use your abs to raise your upper body as high as you can control without flexing your hips.

*The count is 2 seconds up, pause for 2 seconds, then 4 seconds down. Keep the movement slow and under control.

*Make sure not to pull on your head to raise your upper body. That will take pressure off your abs where it belongs and place it on your biceps. Always remember when doing crunches, we're doing abs not arms. Crossing your hands over your chest might help.

*Remember to keep all joints other than your spine stable. Avoid flexing your hip or neck.

*Do as many as you can without losing form.

Starting Position

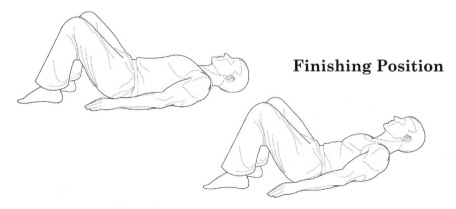

Finishing Position

Crunch (Variation)

There are many ways to vary this exercise in order to hit the muscles in a different way.

One variation involves putting the soles of your feet flat against a wall.

*Your legs should be high enough to form a 90 percent angle.

*The count is 2-2-4. Keep the movement slow and under control.

*Remember not to pull on your head

*Do as many as you can without losing form.

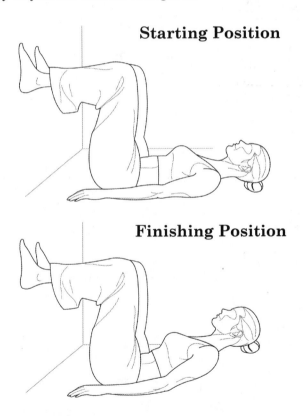

Starting Position

Finishing Position

Every time you contract your abs the opposing muscle group, your lower back muscles, are stretched. That makes crunches an effective lower back stretch in addition to strengthening your abs.

Reverse Crunch

This is another way to effectively develop your abs. Lie down on the mat with your knees bent. Take a deep breath, then as you exhale, use your abdominals to raise your lower body towards your upper body.

*Raise your lower body as high as you can control. Remember that this is a small movement. Too much movement means you're moving something that you shouldn't.

*Remember not to use momentum or to flex your hips.

*Don't tense your leg muscles, keep them relaxed.

*Do as many as you can without losing form.

Starting Position

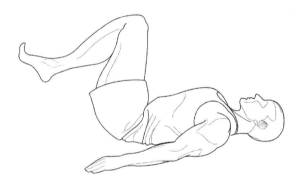

Finishing Position

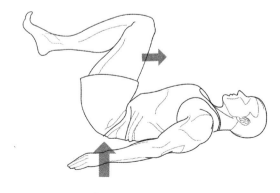

Core

The Plank

The starting position for this exercise is on your elbows and knees. Take a deep breath then as you exhale, draw your navel back towards your spine as you elevate onto your elbows and toes. This change in abdominal position is called the "draw-in maneuver" and should be maintained throughout the exercise.

*Don't allow your lower back to cave-in.

*Hold for 10 seconds.

*Repeat four times.

Starting Position

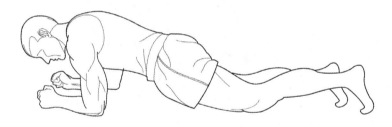

Finishing Position

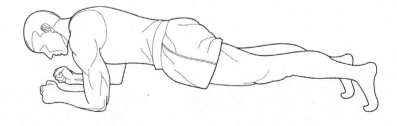

Stability Ball push-ups

Here the goal is to do a traditional push-up with good, solid form. The purpose of the stability ball is to provide an unstable surface. This challenges the postural muscles, which don't normally have to work very hard, by forcing them to stabilize the movement. As you advance you can use two stability balls, one supporting each hand. This adds an extra variable to cope with, thus providing a greater challenge with additional benefit.

Another option is to use a foam roll. These are used for self-myofascial release and are common in most quality gyms. The longer ones give you a wide variety of hand placement options and since they are round, they force you to control their tendency to roll, much as a stability ball would.

Starting Position

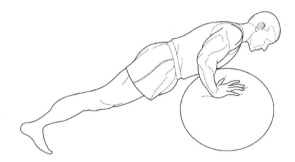

Finishing Position

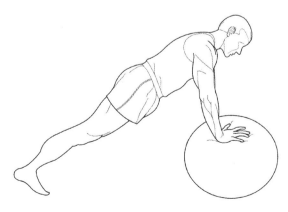

Bridging

Lie down on an exercise mat with your knees bent and your feet flat on the floor. Draw in, squeeze your glutes and push through your heels to elevate yourself into the position shown below. Make sure not to let your abs protrude or your lower back cave in.

*Hold for 10 seconds.

*Repeat four times.

Starting Position

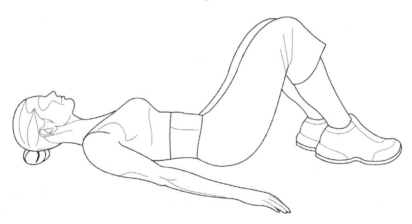

Finishing Position

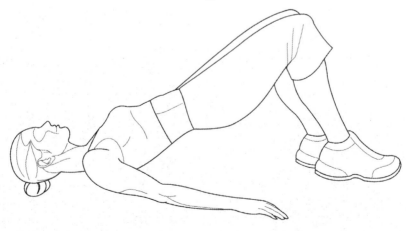

Lower Body

Quadriceps/ Hamstrings

The Squat (Straight Bar)

Stand with your feet hip width apart, pointing forward and the bar resting on the base of your neck. Take a deep breath, then begin to flex your knees and hips. Continue your descent until your thighs are parallel to the floor. Slowly return to starting position.

*Keep your feet pointed forward and your spine neutral; focus your eyes straight ahead.

*Keep your chest up and out.

*Balance yourself over the middle of your feet.

*Don't let your knees move in or out as they extend.

*Don't let your knees move beyond your toes as you descend.

*Make sure not to lean forward and not to let your heels rise off the floor.

*This exercise can also be done using dumbbells.

Starting/Finishing Position   Mid-Position

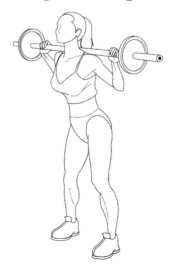
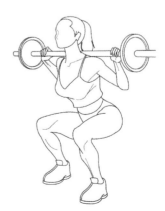

The Leg Press (Machine)

Assume a position with your hips, butt and back pressed evenly against their respective pads. Your feet should be placed on the platform hip width apart and pointed forward. Grasp the handles and extend your knees so that you can remove the machine's support mechanism. Take a deep breath, and lower the platform until your thighs are parallel with the back support. As you exhale, push up through your heels and extend your knees.

*Don't lock your knees at the top of the movement.

*Grasp the machine's hand supports throughout the exercise.

*Always replace the support mechanism before exiting the machine.

Starting/Finishing Position

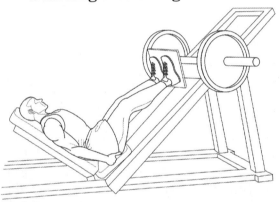

Mid-Position

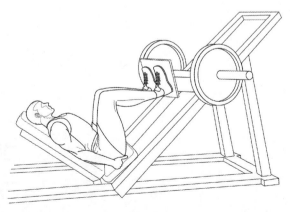

Calves

Calf Raises (Free Weights)

Place your toes on something about three inches high, such as a piece of wood.

Take a deep breath, then as you exhale, draw your navel back towards your spine and rise up onto your toes.

Slowly return to starting position.

Starting Position   **Finishing Position**

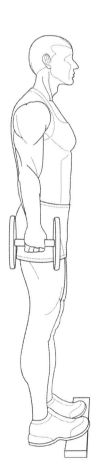 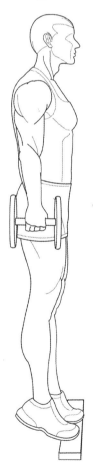

Calf Raises (Leg Press Machine)

Sit comfortably on a leg press machine with the balls of your feet on the platform, about shoulder width apart. Take a deep breath, then as you exhale, point your toes forward, flexing your ankle.

*Don't lock your knees.

*Keep only the balls of your feet on the platform.

*It's a small movement so resist the urge to rush the movement speed.

Starting Position   **Finishing Position**

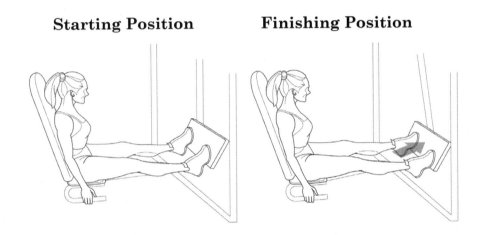

Suggested Reading

Essentials of Strength Training and Conditioning by Thomas R. Baechle, Editor (Human Kinetics Publishers, 2nd edition, July 2000)

Integrated Strength Training by Micheal Clark, CEO of the National Academy of Sports Medicine (NASM)

"The human body was designed to walk, run
or stop; it wasn't built for coasting."
—Cullen Hightower, salesman, author

"For the average person, working out 20 to 30 minutes,
vigorously, three or five times a week, that's good."
—Fitness Guru Jack LaLanne

26 | 6:55 p.m.
Will You Do Cardio?

The fact that good cardiovascular fitness improves both the length and quality of your life is no longer news. According to a study of 45,000 men done by the Harvard University School of Public Health, those who ran for at least an hour each week reduced their risk of death from heart disease by 42 percent. In spite of this, many men I know neglect this important component of their fitness routine in favor of some extra time spent strength training. I have been in and out of countless gyms over the past thirty years. Many of them had lines waiting for the four flat benches, people pacing impatiently by the three squat racks and cobwebs hanging off the one lonely treadmill. Putting only part of a puzzle together should never be your goal. The puzzle that is your health needs to include this crucial piece.

There are several factors to consider when deciding on an endurance training program. They include duration, frequency, mode and intensity. Let's look at each.

Duration

Duration refers to how long an exercise session should last. The minimum recommendation for cardio is 15 to 20 minutes, and is a good choice for those beginning an exercise program. For more experienced exercisers, cardio duration usually ranges between 15 minutes and one hour, though considerably longer sessions are not uncommon, depending on the goal.

Frequency

Frequency refers to how often you exercise. The minimum recommendation for cardio is three to five times a week. For sedentary individuals who are beginning an exercise program, two to three times a week is a sensible place to start. While some people choose to do cardio daily, they risk overtraining which can do more harm than good.

Mode

Mode refers to which exercise is chosen. There are many options, each with their own advantages and disadvantages. Some of the most popular are listed below along with what separates them from the competition.

Walking:

Advantages: For those starting from a low level of fitness, walking is an excellent jumping off point. Studies have shown that walking reduces knee pain in those suffering from osteoarthritis. This type of exercise is low impact and accessible to anyone at almost anytime.

Disadvantages: If you have not done any exercise in a long time, any form of activity will provide cardiovascular benefit, walking included. However, if you are a regular exerciser, or your body adapts to your new walking routine, then walking will provide minimal cardiovascular benefit. Additional benefit can be attained by manipulating the variables, such as picking up the pace or walking uphill. There is no substantial gain in muscular strength.

Elliptical Machine:

Advantages: These machines, which first made the scene in the mid-90s, are now standard equipment in most gyms. According to Dr. Joseph Mercola, author of *Dr. Mercola's Total Health Program*, the number of people using elliptical machines increased from 2.4 million in 1997 to 6.2 million in 2000. Ellipticals can give you a quality workout that is low impact. The moving handles require synchronized movements of the upper and lower body, thereby improving coordination. Keep in mind that the coordination demands are greatly diminished when the stationary handgrips are used, rather than the moving handles.

Disadvantages: In spite of their increasing popularity these machines are not yet available in some gyms. While many manufacturers claim that these machines burn far more calories than a treadmill, a study done by the University of Mississippi found those claims to be inaccurate.

Treadmill/Running:

Advantages: Possibly the most practical form of exercise. A running track is accessible to most people and virtually every gym has a treadmill. Numerous muscle groups receive adequate training from this type of exercise.

Disadvantages: Running, even under optimal conditions, is harder on the joints than some of the other options available to you. Particularly at risk are the knees and back, contraindicating running for those with a history of problems in those areas.

Cycling:

Advantages: A great way to strengthen your quadriceps. The varied terrain and scenery helps to keep the experience from growing stale. Not a bad way to combine exercise with doing your chores.

Disadvantages: Can aggravate certain knee injuries. The cost and storage space required to own a bike is a consideration. Some weather conditions including rain, snow and wind can make this form of exercise impractical. Watch out for traffic which in a split second can turn the aging debate into a non-issue.

Stationary Bike:

Advantages: Still great for the quads and cardiovascular system without needing to worry about good weather, wide open spaces or traffic.

Disadvantages: Can aggravate certain knee injuries. Unless there's something good on TV, there is not much of a view. It's hard to make a stop at the bank on a stationary bike.

*Special note for those with back problems: Try a recumbent bike. Exercising in a reclining position takes much of the pressure off your back, making it a safer and healthier choice. The degree to which these cycles recline varies greatly and can be tailored to the needs of the individual.

Rowing:

Advantages: Aids in developing a high degree of aerobic fitness as well as muscular strength and endurance. Rowing is also a great way to develop coordinated movements of the upper and lower body.

Disadvantages: This type of equipment is unavailable to many. It can also take a while to get this more complex motion to the point where it's smooth and synchronized.

Upper Body Crank Machine (UBC):

Advantages: This machine allows you to get a satisfactory cardiovascular workout using only the muscles of your upper body, a plus for those with serious lower body musculoskeletal conditions.

Disadvantages: Only certain muscle groups benefit from this type of equipment. Assuming your decision is the result of physical limitations that make this choice appropriate, the positives clearly outweigh the negatives.

Aerobics Class:

Advantages: Statistics show that over 60 percent of new exercisers quit within the first six weeks after beginning a new program. The fun and sense of camaraderie that people derive from taking part in group fitness classes can help keep you in the gym.

Disadvantages: Since people are working with others of widely varying fitness levels, they may be inclined to work too hard or not hard enough, thus creating the potential for this form of exercise to be either risky or ineffective.

Stair Climbing/Stair-Climber:

Advantages: A great workout for all the muscles of your lower body. Also, since we often need to climb stairs in the course of our daily life, a little conditioning of the muscles required is a pretty good idea. Those trapped with me in New York's blackout of 2003 either benefited from having climbed stairs regularly or wished that they had.

Disadvantages: Many people have very poor posture when using these machines. If you find yourself leaning forward and dropping your head, straighten up! If not, you may be doing your back and neck more harm than good.

Swimming:

Advantages: Swimming is less stressful on the joints than many other types of exercise, a plus for individuals with chronic orthopedic problems as well as anyone with a recent musculoskeletal injury.

Disadvantages: A primary function of cardiovascular exercise is to elevate the heart rate. The prone position of swimmers, combined with the pool's relatively cool environment, works to suppress your heart rate.

Other Fitness Options

Some people don't like traditional, gym-oriented modes of exercise. If this sounds like you, but your goal is to exercise your way to a more youthful, vibrant life, keep in mind that a number of other fitness options exist. Several of the best and most popular are listed below.

Pilates:

Initially called Controlology by its originator Joseph Pilates, this exercise system now bears his name. Developed in the 1920s as a method of rehabilitation, Pilates has grown into one of today's most popular fitness trends. It is made up of over 500 exercises divided into programs for beginner, intermediate and advanced levels. Many exercises require no equipment while others make use of elaborate devices with names like the Universal Reformer and the Wunda Chair.

Advantages: Great for developing flexibility, core strength and better balance. Balance is particularly important as we age since it reduces the risk of falling. For many techniques little equipment is necessary. Also, since it is trendy, finding a class is easy.

Disadvantages: Lacks substantial cardiovascular benefit; requires a qualified instructor and some equipment.

Yoga:

Yoga is a method of physical, mental and spiritual training dating back thousands of years. Developed in India, yoga uses breathing exercises combined with a series of poses or asanas to develop the life force, referred to by the Sanskrit word Prana.

Advantages: The body will benefit from substantial gains in flexibility and balance. In addition, yoga is one of the best forms of exercise for the mind and spirit. I have heard it said that while Pilates trains the body, yoga trains the mind. According to instructor Anne Taylor, yoga can be used to treat emotional problems like anxiety and depression. Ms. Taylor states, "Yoga can relax both the mind and body."

Disadvantages: Yoga is not as efficient a method of weight loss as one might think. The American Council on Exercise (ACE), estimates that an hour long yoga class burns only about 144 calories, less than many other forms of exercise. While yoga has the image of a safe method of fitness, this is not always true. When polled, chiropractors revealed that as many patients came to them with injuries suffered doing yoga as did so from injuries related to weight training. Even more disturbing is that those numbers are on the rise. This fact can be attributed to students trying to go beyond their limits, often without proper supervision, rather than any problem inherent to yoga itself. Some styles of yoga lack substantial cardiovascular benefit.

Types of Yoga
There are many styles to choose from, each with its own focus. The four primary types of yoga are: Karma, Bhakthi, Raja and Gyana, also known as Jhana. Within the Raja style, there is a subdivision called Hatha, which uses postures as a point of meditation. Hatha is considered the most popular style of yoga in America today.

Poses/Asanas
A typical yoga class is about an hour and a half long and is made up of between ten and thirty or more asanas, depending on the style. Iyenger, a very detail oriented style, has fewer poses which are held from one to five minutes each. By contrast, Vinyasa, a more power oriented style, can have thirty or more poses in a single class.

Bikram Yoga
The brainchild of Calcutta-born Bikram Choudhury, the unique feature of this style is that it is performed in a room that has been heated to just over 100 degrees. According to instructor Viraj Santini, this intense isometric workout is especially popular with men, particularly athletes, and was recommended by fitness guru Joe Weider in his book, *Ultimate Bodybuilding*. The classes are uniform, each consisting of 26 poses.

Advantages: The extreme temperatures facilitate flexibility far beyond the individual's normal range of motion. According to Mr. Santini, the extreme temperatures leave you, "Feeling like melted butter."

Disadvantages: Exercising in conditions of extreme heat can be dangerous, especially for those who are out of shape or suffer from heart disease or respiratory problems.

Want More Info?
For more information *Yoga Journal* has an excellent website. Visit them at: www.yogajournal.com.

For more info on Bikram Yoga, visit their website at: www.bikramyoga.com.

Martial Arts:

There are many styles from many places but all share similar goals; to strengthen the participant physically, mentally and spiritually. Be aware that some schools include full-contact sparring, which on occasion can result in injury. While this risk should not be ignored, most styles teach viable self-defense techniques that can be lifesavers. For those seeking only cardiovascular benefit, training without contact is also available.

Choosing a Martial Arts School

Your health, both physical and mental, can benefit greatly from choosing the right martial arts school. The wrong choice can result in injury or a waste of your valuable time. There are several points to consider for those who would like to choose wisely.

First, you must decide which style is right for you. Someone who is powerfully built might choose Shotokan Karate, while those who like a fast paced system based on flexibility might enjoy Wing Chun, a method studied by the late Bruce Lee. If strategy is your game then Seven Star Praying Mantis is an excellent choice. If you prefer a softer touch and a slower pace, then Tai Chi might be the way to go, while those who want something more gymnastic might prefer Brazilian Capoeira.

Another consideration is the quality of instruction. No matter how badly you want to study Eagle Claw Kung Fu, if the school is not of a high caliber, then you are unlikely to benefit from attending its classes. Always observe a class before registering. By watching what you're in for, you can save yourself some time and money. Beware of schools where the same instructor teaches many different styles. We've all heard the expression, "Jack of all trades, master of none." Make sure Jack isn't instructing you in Judo between teaching Tae Kwon Do to one class and Kendo to another.

Finally there are logistical concerns. Two key factors are location and class schedule. If the classes are at a time and place that is inconvenient, chances are good that you will quit before gaining much from the experience.

Sports (Tennis, Soccer, Racquetball, etc.):

Advantage: Since they are playing a game, many people enjoy this type of exercise more than the monotony of other methods.

Disadvantages: This is not nearly as structured an activity as the others mentioned, making results harder to predict and intensity harder to monitor. Since movements are more random, and body contact possible, there is an increased risk of injury.

Dance:

Advantages: For those who suffer from back pain, some studies have shown that many popular styles of dance help to alleviate the problem. The fact that these art forms are often done for pleasure as well as fitness increases the likelihood that participants will stick with the program. They also fit well within the exercise community's current movement towards coordinated, full body forms of exercise.

Disadvantages: While a sedentary person will benefit aerobically from almost any type of physical activity, someone who exercises regularly, and is in good cardiovascular condition, may not find many styles of dance to be a strenuous workout. Most styles of dance offer limited strength-training benefit. Since dance is often fairly freeform, developing a precise program that can be carefully monitored can be difficult. Some styles can also be hard on the knees and ankles.

A Final Word

Keep in mind that whatever mode you choose, it should be varied periodically. Doing so will prevent an adaptation to the stimulus that may eventually cause your progress to grind to a halt. Doing the same exact workout for years at a time may be comfortable. Still, most exercisers want more than comfort, they want results. Remember, if you want to progress, challenge yourself!

Intensity

Intensity can be defined as how hard you want your heart to work. Since working too hard can be dangerous, and not working hard enough can give you too little benefit, this is perhaps the most crucial of the four criteria.

Choosing Exercise Intensity

There are numerous methods, some quite precise, others more subjective, used to make this determination. We'll look at several of the more popular ones while weighing their pros and cons.

Heart Rate Reserve

Here we take the number 220, subtract the person's age and divide the remainder by between 50 and 90 percent. The percentage we choose depends on the individual's fitness level and number of recognized coronary risk factors. The seven risk factors, as determined by the American College of Sports Medicine (ACSM), are listed below.

Coronary Artery Disease Risk Factors*

The American College of Sports Medicine (ACSM) has identified seven coronary risk factors that need to be considered when designing an exercise program. They include:

1. Family history	Myocardial infarction, coronary revascularization, or sudden death before 55 years of age in father or other male first-degree relative, or before 65 years of age in mother or other female first-degree relative
2. Cigarette smoking	Current cigarette smoker or those who quit within the previous 6 months
3. Hypertension	Systolic blood pressure $\geq$140 mm Hg or diastolic $\geq$90 mm Hg, confirmed by measurements on at least two separate occasions, or on antihypertensive medication
4. Dyslipidemia	Low-density lipoprotein (LDL) cholesterol >130 mg$\cdot$dL^{-1} (3.4 mmol$\cdot$L^{-1}) or high-density lipoprotein (HDL) cholesterol <40 mg$\cdot$dL^{-1} (1.03 mmol$\cdot$L^{-1}), or on lipid-lowering medication. If total serum cholesterol is all that is available use >200 mg$\cdot$dL^{-1} (5.2 mmo$\cdot$L^{-1}) rather than low-density lipoprotein (LDL) >130 mg$\cdot$dL^{-1}
5. Impaired fasting glucose	Fasting blood glucose $\geq$100 mg$\cdot$dL^{-1} (5.6 mmo$\cdot$L^{-1}) confirmed by measurements on at least two separate occasions
6. Obesity	Body mass index >30 kg$\cdot$m^{-2} or Waist girth >102 cm for men and >88 cm for women or Waist/hip ratio $\geq$0.95 for men and $\geq$0.86 for women

7. Sedentary lifestyle   Persons not participating in a regular exercise program or not meeting the minimal physical activity recommendations from the U.S. Surgeon General's Report

They also list one negative risk factor which reduces the risk of heart disease:

1. High-serum HDL   >60 mg•dL^{-1} (1.6 mmol•L^{-1})
   cholesterol

*ACSM'S Guidelines for Exercise Testing and Prescription 7ed ET AL ACSM "2007;22:TB2.2"

Important

Men over 45, women over 55, and all those who meet the threshold for two or more risk factors are classified as being in the moderate risk category. It is highly recommended that these individuals receive a doctor's okay before beginning any exercise program. The same is true for anyone with a history of cardiovascular, pulmonary or metabolic disease.

Examples

Example 1) Let's assume we have a thirty-year-old woman with none of the seven risk factors. We determine that we want her to work at an intensity of 80 percent. We take 220, subtract 30 and divide the remainder by .80.

Example #1

220
-30
190
x.80
152

Using this method we have determined that we want this individual to exercise at a heart rate no higher than 152 beats per minute.

Example 2) Now let's take a fifty-year-old man. Men over 45 are considered to be in the moderate risk category, so age becomes a factor. In this case, our friend is also a smoker. As a result, we want to start him at a lower intensity, about 60 percent. Here we take 220, subtract 50 and divide the remainder by .60.

Example #2

220
-50
170
x.60
102

Using this method we have determined that we want this individual to exercise at a heart rate no higher than 102 beats per minute.

Percentage of Heart Rate Reserve (Karvonen Formula)

This is another heart-rate-based method of calculating exercise intensity. It varies from the previous method by adding resting heart rate into the equation. To illustrate this method let us assume that the woman in our first example has a resting heart rate of 70, and the man in example two has one of 80. Here is how this method would play out:

Example #1

220	
-30	
190	
-70	Resting Heart Rate
120	
x.80	
96	
+70	Resting Heart Rate
166	

Using this method we have determined that we want this individual to exercise at a heart rate no higher than 166 beats per minute.

Example #2

220	
-50	
170	
-80	Resting Heart Rate
90	
x.60	
54	
+80	Resting Heart Rate
134	

Using this method we have determined that we want this individual to exercise at a heart rate no higher than 134 beats per minute.

Note that the target heart rates that result from this formula are higher, making this method riskier than using heart rate reserve. As a result, it should only be used in conjunction with a more subjective method, like the Talk Test or Rating of Perceived Exertion.

Talk Test

This is a popular, totally subjective way of measuring exercise intensity. Here you try having a conversation while exercising. If you can do so comfortably, then chances are good that you are working at a safe level.

Rating Of Perceived Exertion (RPE)

Developed in the 1950s by Swedish physiologist Dr. Gunner Borg, this is another subjective way of measuring exercise intensity. The individual rates the difficulty of their activity on a scale of six to twenty. It has been found that those choosing eight usually have heart rates around eighty, while those who select twelve have hearts that are beating about one hundred and twenty times per minute. A newer model was developed using a scale of one to ten. While simpler to use, it was still found to be an effective tool in gauging how hard a person was working. This method, while not as scientific as others, tends to be fairly accurate. It is a good choice when used in conjunction with more scientific methods.

A Word of Caution

It is crucial that individuals taking medication to control high blood pressure do not choose their exercise intensity solely by a heart rate based method. These medications lower heart rate artificially, making the readout on a monitoring device deceptive. Beta blockers are a particular concern. It is therefore necessary for individuals who are taking these medications to factor in a more subjective method such as the talk test or RPE.

Equipment

Heart Rate Monitors

These handy devices enable the user to get a steady, dependable readout of their heart rate just by glancing at their wrist. They usually consist of two components. One is strapped around your chest and reads your heart rate then relays the information to a wrist-worn receiver that displays it. There are numerous models from which to choose, many offering additional features such as average heart rate and exercise duration. Keep in mind that the batteries don't last forever and can be expensive to replace. Perhaps the best known brand is Polar. You can check their website located at www.polarca.com and browse through currently available models.

Pedometer

When walking is your mode of exercise, a pedometer is an excellent tool. It counts each step, enabling you to keep track of your progress. Perhaps the highest-rated model is the Yamax Digiwalker SW-200. It offers a high degree of accuracy at a reasonable price, generally about $20.00.

Footwear

What Shoe Is Right For Me?
Over 43 million Americans have trouble with their feet, a problem that can often be traced to shoes that don't fit properly. The right shoe depends on individual need. Some are made for specific activities such as running, tennis or walking. There are also shoes with more padding for those who are overweight, elderly or have orthopedic problems.

When shopping for athletic shoes, it is important to find the proper fit. Ideally you should have about a half inch of space in the toe. As for the heel, it should fit snugly so that it does not move when you do. When trying on athletic shoes, remember to wear the type of socks that you'll have on when you exercise. Doing so insures that your only surprise will be how fast you run.

It is also important to choose the right shoe for the activity in which you plan to engage. If you intend to do some running, then get a flexible shoe with extra padding. If walking is your game, then go for something stiffer.

A word to the wise: If you'd like to get the most for your money consider outlet stores. They often get the same products six months after their debut at the more fashionable shoe emporiums, and sell them at a substantial discount.

Running On Empty: When to Change Your Running Shoes

Sneakers that once fit properly may no longer do so. This is often the result of normal wear and tear. Since one hour of strenuous exercise subjects your feet to about a million pounds of pressure, your athletic shoes need to be checked frequently to make sure that they are still up to par. A good rule of thumb is to replace them every 400 miles of use. While this is good in theory, not everyone moves the same way. As a result, it is important to regularly check your heels and soles for signs of excessive wear.

Don't Ignore Mother Nature

Research reported in the September/October issue of *ACE Fitness Matters* claimed that people who live in humid climates are far less active. The study compared data compiled by the Centers for Disease Control and Prevention (CDC), with information provided by 255 of the nation's weather stations. It reported that only between 30 and 38 percent of US residents living in those climates received the 30 or more minutes of moderate daily activity that the CDC recommends. It's important to stay active even when living in weather conditions that make it less comfortable. There are however, some important steps to take to make those conditions both safer and more tolerable.

Heat and Humidity: Wear loose-fitting clothing. This will keep perspiration away from your skin, allowing it to evaporate. Dark colors absorb heat, so the ones you choose should be light. If the sun is strong, wear a hat. Water requirements are a major concern under these conditions. Be aware of fluid intake and make sure to rehydrate at regular intervals.

Cold: Cold can be just as damaging as heat. Make sure to dress in layers. Keeping your head, hands and ears covered is also advisable. In addition, cold weather causes the kidneys to increase their production of urine, making it important to monitor fluid intake to avoid dehydration.

High Altitude: For those unaccustomed to this type of environment, exercise intensity must be carefully monitored and probably reduced. The air at altitudes of 8,000 feet or higher has significantly less oxygen than many people are used to and can cause symptoms that include headaches, dizziness and irritability. The good news is that the symptoms are usually temporary. The period of time required to adapt to such surroundings is approximately two to five weeks depending on the altitude.

Interval Training

This variable in aerobic fitness training involves measured periods of high intensity, immediately followed by periods of low intensity. The intervals are then repeated several times. A good example would be running for three minutes then walking for two. You would then repeat this cycle as many times as necessary to achieve the desired exercise duration. Interval training enables new exercisers to work their way into shape gradually, while at the same time providing variety for those who have been training for an extended period of time. There is also a variation called Fartlik training, where the intervals are not measured but are instead determined by the way the individual feels.

Cool Down

After your workout a cool down is highly recommended. It allows your body to gradually return to its pre-exercise state as blood is allowed to slowly leave the extremities and return to the body's core. A cool down is especially important for anyone with a history of heart problems. Certain hormones related to exercise are at higher than normal levels following a vigorous exercise session. A gradual cool down helps prevent a disturbance in cardiac rhythm.

Suggested Reading

The Running Times Guide to Breakthrough Running by Gordon Bakoulis, Editor-in-Chief (Human Kinetics, May 2000)

*"You can't help getting older,
but you don't have to get old."*
—George Burns

Section IV

AFTER YOUR WORKOUT: LIVING IT UP, THEN WINDING DOWN

"Tell me what you eat, and I will tell you what you are."
—Anthelme Brillat-Savarin

27 | 7:20 p.m. What is Your Second Snack?

Workout Day Snacking

You have just finished your workout. Exercise depletes your muscles' stores of glycogen, the form in which your body stores carbohydrates. In spite of the undeserved bad rap that carbs have been given, they are your body's preferred fuel source and need to be replenished. The American College of Sports Medicine recommends consuming between 200 and 400 calories from carbohydrate sources immediately following exercise. Because of this, having a carbohydrate-rich snack shortly after your workout is an excellent idea. Something with a high glycemic index is recommended to help resynthesize glycogen back into your muscles. Good choices include a box of raisins, some carrots or a baked potato— hold the butter and salt.

Juicing

Another option is to dust off your juicer. When I juice regularly, my health is better and I'm more resistant to exercise-related soreness.

Here are a few of my favorite recipes:

Fruit Based

Recipe 1) One-half a pineapple: Pineapple contains bromalain, a natural anti-inflammatory.

1 orange: Peel but leave as much of the pith, white material between the fruit and the peel, as possible. It's high in bioflavonoids, substances that work synergistically with vitamin C to repair tissues.

1 grapefruit: Peel the same as above.

Additional ingredients: A handful of strawberries, grapes, cranberries (when in season), an apple, some cantaloupe or watermelon.

Recipe 2) 2 Apples: Peeled, seeds removed

Half a lemon: Peeled

8oz. of water: Filtered or bottled

This combination offers a carbohydrate boost plus plenty of water to rehydrate you. In addition, drinking fresh lemon juice is a great way to detoxify the body.

Vegetable Based

1 bag of carrots: Remove the top and bottom and wash thoroughly. Do not peel.

1 apple: Peeled, seeds removed

Those with sports-related inflammation of tendons or muscles might benefit from adding cucumbers or peppers to their juice. Both contain a large quantity of silicon, a mineral that reduces inflammation. Silicon has also demonstrated the ability to rejuvenate tired muscles.

Additional ingredients: Most any vegetable that's healthy to eat is also healthy to juice. Here are a few you might consider experimenting with: asparagus, tomatoes, broccoli, celery and cauliflower. Some vegetables are healthy, but their effect on your system is powerful. While you can benefit from including these in the juices you prepare, they should only make up a small percentage of its total volume. These vegetables include: garlic, onions, parsley and beets. Also consider adding a quarter- inch piece of peeled ginger.

A Few Juicing Dos and Don'ts

*Do remove all pits, though seeds, with the exception of apple seeds, can be placed in the juicer. Apple seeds contain trace amounts of cyanide and should not be ingested.

*Do wash all produce thoroughly before juicing. This is especially important when using produce that is not organically grown.

*Do drink the juice as soon as possible. The vitamins and minerals that are abundant in fresh fruit and vegetable juice begin lose potency as soon as the juice is made. If you choose to store your juice, make sure that it is refrigerated in an airtight container. Drink stored juice within 48 hours.

*Don't load up *too* heavily on greens. If too high a percentage of your vegetable juice comes from greens, (broccoli, spinach, peppers, etc.), it may upset your stomach. Limit the percentage of your vegetable juice that is made from green vegetables to 25 percent of the total volume.

*Don't mix vegetables with fruit. This rule is by no means absolute, but since your body handles fruits and vegetables differently, doing so could cause some digestive problems. Mixing the two may also result in some unfortunate tasting juice. Exceptions to this rule are apples, which mix nicely with any vegetable combination, and tomatoes, peppers and cucumbers, which are actually fruit.

*Don't bother juicing bananas. The low water content will result in no juice as well as one messy banana.

Want More Info?

Below are several books I own on juicing. They explain the concept in detail as well as offering a vast array of recipes to suit any taste.

The Juiceman's Power of Juicing by Jay Kordich (Morrow Cookbooks, 1st edition, April 20, 1992)

Juicing For Life by Cherie Calbom and Maureen Keane (Avery, November 1, 1991)

The Juicing Book by Stephen Blauer (Avery, May 1, 1989)

Non-Workout Day Snacking

As mentioned earlier, it is unlikely that you will workout every day. On days when you do not exercise you can have your second snack earlier, around 3:00 or 3:30, if the work day allows. If that is not possible, grab something after work, around 5:30 or 6:00. This will space your meals out better, allowing you to maximize the benefits of the five-meal-a-day plan. Your snack choices on those days include all the options listed in this chapter as well as any from snack number one, as detailed in chapter 18.

A Final Word on Snacking

A word of caution when it comes to snacking, five small meals mean just that—small. Don't replace three 700 calorie meals with five 700 calorie meals. If you do, the scale will not be your friend.

"Let food be your medicine and medicine be your food."
—Hippocrates

28 8 p.m. What Will You Have For Dinner?

While many of us skip breakfast, we usually work in dinner. This is a meal where we tend to poison ourselves with tons of salt, fat, cholesterol and other goodies that may cut our dinner-eating future short. Make sure that your meal consists of a sensible balance of nutrients and keep portion sizes reasonable. Some healthy choices for both eating in and out are listed below.

Eating In

General Guidelines

*Start with a salad: Eating a variety of vegetables on a regular basis can add years to your life. In addition to their vast nutritional value, the high fiber content of green, leafy vegetables will fill you up, decreasing your desire to overeat. Include broccoli whenever possible and top with parsley or sprouts. Remember to keep the dressing to a minimum.

*Your freezer is your friend: Preparing healthy meals in advance will cut down on unhealthy meals eaten out or ordered in. You can cook dinner for the week and freeze it. Soups are a particularly good choice. Make a pot of split pea on Sunday and enjoy it throughout the week.

*Veggies on the side: Most experts agree that approximately 50 percent of your diet should be comprised of fresh fruits and vegetables. One of the best choices is asparagus. These tasty green spears are rich in vitamin K, which helps to build strong bones and prevent heart disease. Asparagus is also high in glutathione, a compound that fights cancer and bolsters the immune system. In addition, its extremely high folate content helps protect against age-related memory loss. Other great choices include broccoli, cauliflower and spinach.

*Top with chives: Chives are a pungent plant that is high in vitamin C, folic acid and potassium, nutrients often harmed during cooking. By adding chives to the dishes you've prepared, some of those lost nutrients can be restored.

*Eat "Healthy": The word healthy, when listed on a food label, is more than just marketing. For a manufacturer to use this term, certain minimum nutritional requirements must be met. These include maximum sodium content of 360 mg for individual foods, while meals and main dishes cannot exceed 480 mg.

*Cut the cake: Rather than stuffing yourself with cake filled with sugar and chemicals, why not finish with something healthy? Remember the fruit bowl Aunt Jenny gave you for Christmas and how you couldn't figure out what to do with it? Why not fill it with fruit? Consider a combination of strawberries, blueberries and raspberries. They provide you with the sweet taste you crave and the nutrients you need.

Shopping Tip

Don't shop when you're hungry. Doing so will often lead to poor decision making. Make a list of problem foods *before* you get to the supermarket. By referring to it as you shop you can keep the toxins in your kitchen to a minimum.

Recipe Ideas

Work days are long and getting longer, as are commutes. This leads many people to abandon healthy meals that require some preparation in favor of heavily processed foods that can be popped into the microwave. Below are a few ideas that will make your meal healthy without taking all night to prepare.

A tofu and vegetable stir fry: This tasty, healthful dish is easy to prepare, ideal for kitchen klutzes like me. Use low fat tofu whenever possible to keep the calorie count in check.

Grilled chicken with a sweet potato and a side of quinoa: Grilled food is much healthier than fried food and lean meats like chicken are far superior to beef. Quinoa, classified by the United Nations as a "super crop", surpasses wheat in almost every nutritional category. Sweet potatoes are loaded with vitamin C, potassium and fiber.

Whole-wheat pasta and frozen vegetables: Consider adding a package of frozen vegetables to your pasta. Doing so will enhance both the health benefits and the flavor. This combination is easy to prepare and contains a laundry list of nutrients.

Sautéed shiitake mushrooms over pasta or rice: Few people realize the healing power that lies within these succulent fungi. Shiitake mushrooms contain a substance called lentinan that has a positive effect on the immune system. Lentinan, a polysaccharide, has also demonstrated anti-tumor activity. Eritadenine, another compound contained in shiitake mushrooms, is helpful in lowering cholesterol levels.

For those who like detailed recipes, here are three borrowed from Dr. Jane Pentz's book, *If You Don't Take Care of Your Body, Where are You Going to Live?* They list exactly what ingredients are involved, as well as detailed instructions on how to prepare them. Here is one fish dish, one poultry and one vegetarian. Enjoy!

Fiesta Pasta & Tuna Salad

Tricolor corkscrew pasta and tuna provide a colorful, festive, cool salad dish with carbs, protein and low fat. Prepare and cook in 30 minutes!

Serves 4

Ingredients

8	ounces tricolor corkscrew pasta
16	ounces green beans, trimmed and cut into 2-inch pieces
1	medium red onion, thinly sliced (about 1 cup)
$2/3$	cup reduced-fat Italian salad dressing
$1/4$	cup chopped fresh parsley
$1/4$	cup chopped fresh basil
1	cup cherry tomatoes cut in half
2	cans (6 $1/8$ ounces each) tuna packed in water, drained and flaked

Fresh basil sprigs for garnish

Preparation
Cook pasta according to package directions, but eliminate salt. About 7 minutes before pasta is done, add green beans to pot. Remove pot from heat and add onion. Drain in colander and rinse under cold water. Drain again.

While pasta mixture is draining, combine dressing, parsley, and chopped basil in large serving bowl. Mix well.

Add pasta mixture to dressing mixture. Add tomatoes and tuna. Toss to coat. Garnish with basil sprigs and serve.

Hint
This recipe provides a complete meal.

Per Serving

Calories	361 (10% from fat)	Fat	4g
Carbohydrates	54g	Protein	27g

Sue's Grilled Chicken & Broccoli in Red Sauce

Grilled chicken in tomato sauce with fresh vegetables gives this healthy dish a unique flavor.

Serves 4

Ingredients

1	teaspoon olive oil
1	pound boneless, skinless chicken grilled and sliced into strips
1	28 ounce can No Salt Added Whole tomatoes undrained & chopped
4-6	plum tomatoes coarsely chopped
2	cups broccoli florets
1	cup fresh sliced mushrooms
3	tablespoons fresh chopped parsley
4-5	cloves fresh garlic thinly sliced
8	black olives sliced in half

Fresh basil, chopped
Salt and pepper to taste

Preparation
Combine canned and fresh tomatoes, parsley, salt, and fresh ground pepper in a bowl; set aside. (This can be done several hours ahead.)

Sauté garlic in olive oil until fragrant. Add tomato mixture, bring to a boil.

Add chicken pieces, broccoli, mushrooms, and olives and simmer approximately 15 minutes until vegetables are cooked but still firm.

Serve over pasta, sprinkle with fresh basil.

Try This
Grilled shrimp can be substituted for chicken for a great tasting seafood dinner.

Hint
Here's another great meal that's complete when served over pasta.

Per Serving

Calories	250 (23% from fat)	Fat	6.5g
Carbohydrates	11g	Protein	37g

Sue's Pasta with Roasted Red Pepper Sauce

Roasting peppers takes a little bit of time, but it is well worth it for the flavor! Use roasted peppers on sandwiches too!

Serves 4

Ingredients

1	teaspoon olive oil
2	cups onion, chopped
4	cloves garlic, minced
½	teaspoon fennel seeds, crushed
2	28 ounce cans No-Salt Added whole tomatoes undrained and chopped
1	pound red peppers, roasted and peeled (see directions)
1	pound green peppers, roasted and peeled (see directions)
1	pound yellow peppers, roasted and peeled (see directions)
½	teaspoon salt and fresh ground pepper to taste
½	bunch thinly sliced fresh basil
4	cups cooked pasta

Preparation
Sauté onion, fennel seeds, and garlic in olive oil until tender, about 5 minutes, stirring occasionally.

Add tomatoes, bring to simmer.

Add pepper strips, salt, and pepper, and half of the basil. Simmer on low heat, stirring occasionally, about 45 minutes.

Serve over pasta, sprinkle with remaining basil and fresh grated parmesan cheese.

For Roasting Peppers
Cut peppers in half lengthwise; discard seeds and membranes. Place peppers, skin side up on a foil lined baking sheet, flatten with palm of hand.

Broil (close to heat) until blackened and charred (about 10 minutes).

Place in zip-lock heavy-duty plastic bag, seal and let stand 15 minutes or so. Remove from bag, peel and discard skins.

Hint
Drink a glass of milk to complete this meal.

Per Serving

Calories	271 (16% from fat)	Fat	3g
Carbohydrates	51g	Protein	10g

Eating Out

This can be tricky. Since you're not preparing the food, you don't really know what you're getting. Here are a few tips that can make eating out a healthier and more pleasurable experience.

*Avoid Swordfish: Swordfish steak is a popular dish in many seafood restaurants. Unfortunately swordfish, like shark, is high in mercury. Because of this, intake of swordfish should be kept to a minimum.

*Brown Rice: Choose brown rice over white. Brown rice is high in phosphorous, potassium, iron, thiamin and cancer fighting insoluble fiber. The difference between brown and white rice is the presence of the husks. Once the husks are removed, rice is more aesthetically pleasing, but also loses most of its nutritional value.

*Watch Out for Fancy Restaurants: Rich sauces and other ingredients are involved in making their food both pricey and distinctive; they can damage more than your wallet.

*Bring Your Own Salad Dressing: This can be a nuisance but salad dressing is often one of the unhealthiest items on the menu. Apple cider vinegar is something you can bring with you. If you can't, or prefer not to, consider ordering oil and vinegar dressing, on the side.

*Avoid Fried Foods: These foods have the taste that many people crave but are high in both calories and saturated fat. Opt for meals that are grilled, steamed, broiled or baked. Replace French fries with baked potatoes, hold the butter and salt. While Japanese food is often a healthy choice, remember that tempura is fried.

Dinner Dos:

*Feel Free to Eat Earlier: Having dinner at 8pm fits nicely into our workout-day schedule, since it allows for a small post workout snack and enough time to get to your dinner location. On non-workout days feel free to move your dinner time up, as you did with the time of snack number two. If you snack between 3:00 and 4pm, dinner around 6:00 or 6:30 works well. If you don't snack until 5:30, consider dining around 7:00 or 7:30.

*Work Salmon into Your Diet Several Times a Week: This fatty fish has been touted for its ability to fight heart disease, due largely to its high levels of omega-3 fatty acids. These substances raise your level of high-density lipoproteins (HDL), the so called "friendly fat." HDL fights heart disease by removing cholesterol from the arteries and transporting it to the liver so that it can be eliminated from the body. If you don't like salmon, or if it is not available, mackerel, albacore and herring are other great choices, for the same heart healthy reason. Salmon's high vitamin B6 content makes it an effective weapon in fighting diabetes. The oils in fish also protect your eyes against macular degeneration.

Keep in mind when purchasing salmon fillets that eating wild salmon is far more beneficial to your health than consuming those raised on farms. Farm raised fish are often shot full of antibiotics and frequently contain PCBs, dioxins and other contaminants. In addition, the levels of omega-3 fatty acids are often higher in salmon that are caught in the wild. Since not all salmon that is said to be wild actually is, it is wise to purchase fish that are from Alaska where salmon farming is illegal. To purchase salmon fillets and other quality seafood consider the following source:

Seafood Direct: 1-800-732-1836 www.buyseafooddirect.com

*Take Something Home: Portion sizes in restaurants across America have been growing at a rate only equaled by diner's waistlines. Still, patrons seem only too happy to clean their plates. While doggie bags may not seem stylish, they get you into the habit of not consuming every available morsel. When it comes to cutting back on portion size, Doctor James Dillard agrees, "The only reliable way to extend the lifespan of a mammal is *under-nutrition* without malnutrition. Studies show that if you cut back on 60% of the calories mice eat, they will live almost twice as long with much fewer tumors."

*Eat Less Red Meat: While many people love a thick, juicy steak, red meat increases your risk of many serious health problems. These conditions include:

- Colon Cancer: As verified by a study conducted by The American Cancer Society between 1982 and 2001.

- Rheumatoid Arthritis: According to a study conducted in Britain by Dorothy Pattison, PhD.

- Diabetes: As per findings of the Harvard Medical School, reported in the September 2004 issue of *Diabetes Care*.

*Drink Plenty of Water: It is important to consume plenty of fluids with meals. They aid in the digestive process and increase satiety. For reasons of conservation some restaurants no longer serve water unless you request it. Remember to do so at every meal.

*Ask Questions: "Is this fish cooked in butter?", "Can you leave out the MSG?" Many people are uncomfortable asking questions like those, but being an informed shopper can make a big difference in how healthy your dinner proves to be. Ever hear the expression, "The customer is always right"? Never forget that you're paying for the goods and services that you are receiving and deserve to be treated with courtesy and respect.

Dinner Don'ts:

*Watch Out For Buffets: A very popular concept in many cities is the all- you- can- eat buffet. The problem with offering people all they can eat is that many of them will do just that. Remember that restaurants that serve unlimited quantity often do so at the expense of quality.

*Avoid Processed Foods: The processing involved in preparing many foods kills valuable nutrients and replaces them with harmful chemicals.

*Avoid Canned Foods: Canned foods often contain a great deal of salt. While your body requires only half a gram (500 milligrams) of sodium per day, the average American consumes between 12 and 36 times that amount. Half a can of some popular brands of condensed soup contains half your daily allotment. If you eat canned foods (other than soup) remember to rinse them first. This removes much of the unwanted sodium.

*Avoid Soft Drinks and Desserts: As with lunch, both soda and sugary desserts should be avoided at dinner. Both pour toxic substances into your system that it will have to cope with and try to eliminate.

*Don't Drink Too Much Coffee: While a little coffee is probably not going to do you much harm, remember not to overdo it. According to nutritionist, Linda Feingold, "Many people rely on caffeine for energy instead of food. Caffeinated beverages only provide a false sense of energy that quickly dissipates, leaving you feeling energy-depleted in the end. Only calories can provide true energy for your brain and muscles." Many experts also believe that coffee, especially unfiltered coffee, may contribute to higher levels of cholesterol.

The detrimental effects of coffee are not always the fault of the beverage itself; they may also reflect the substances that we choose to add. Pouring sugar or milk into your cup, or topping it off with whipped cream, can add lots of fat to your drink along with loads of empty calories.

An Interesting Theory

According to Brian Wansink, a researcher at the University of Illinois, dim light does more than set the mood, it may also increase food intake. Dr. Wansink claims that, "Dim light makes you feel uninhibited," thereby causing you to overeat. Keep that in mind during your next candlelit dinner, and make sure an extra helping doesn't leave you too full for romance.

Suggested Reading

Small Changes, Big Results: A 12-Week Action Plan to a Better Life by Ellie Krieger and Kelly James-Enger (Three Rivers Press, Reprint edition, December 27, 2005)

Nutrition for Life by Lisa Hark and Darwin Deen (DK ADULT, January 17, 2005)

Moosewood Restaurant Simple Suppers: Fresh Ideas for the Weeknight Table by Moosewood Collective (Clarkson Potter, October 25, 2005)

Six Arguments for a Greener Diet: How a Plant-based Diet Could Save Your Health and the Environment by Michael F. Jacobson and Center for Science in the Public Interest (Center for Science in the Public Interest, July 31, 2006)

"Alcohol is the anesthesia by which we endure the operation of life."
—Samuel Johnson

29 8 p.m.
Will You Drink Alcohol and if So, How Much?

Answering yes to this question can be a plus or a big minus depending on the type and quantity. It has been accepted by the medical community that one or two drinks per day has health benefits, the best choice being red wine. One drink is defined as 12 ounces of beer, four to five ounces of wine or 1-1¼ ounces of 80 proof distilled liquor. Caution: More than two drinks is a negative, possibly a big one.

Benefits of Moderate Drinking

A Drink a Day Keeps Dementia Away?

Can drinking actually keep your mind sharp? According to *The Nurses' Health Study*, the answer might be yes. They tracked the alcohol consumption of 12,480 female nurses starting in 1980, and evaluated the results between 1995 and 2001. All the participants were 70 to 81 years old at the time of the evaluation, and had been moderate drinkers. The findings, reported on January 20, 2005 in *The New England Journal of Medicine*, might both surprise you and cheer up your favorite bartender. They found that, "Up to one drink per day does not impair cognitive function and may actually decrease the risk of cognitive decline."

Moderate Alcohol Consumption and Heart Disease

There is more good news from the same source. The results of the *Nurse's Health Study* in regard to the risk of heart disease for women between 50 and 70 years of age showed that, "The group who drank three or more drinks per week (one-half of one drink per day) had a 40 percent lower rate of non-fatal heart attacks and arterial disease than the group which did not." It claimed similar results for men. The study stated that there appears to be an ideal "range" for alcohol consumption, one-half of one drink per day for women, and one to two drinks a day for men.

Those looking to drink their way to a healthy heart should consider red wine as their drink of choice. This is due to the well documented link between moderate red wine consumption and a reduced risk of cardiovascular disease. To maximize wine's health benefits, choose those that hail from Sardinia or the southwestern part of France. The seeds and skins of grapes grown in those regions contain high concentrations of oligomeric procyanidins, nutrients thought to protect veins, strengthen capillaries and speed the return of blood to the heart from the lower extremities.

Alcohol and Memory

While many people drink to forget their problems, studies show that moderate alcohol consumption may actually *preserve* your memory. Alcohol has exhibited the ability to prevent blood from clotting, to reduce inflammation and to increase the release of acetylcholine, a neurotransmitter. All of these factors may play a role in preserving memory as we age.

Alcohol and Osteoporosis

There is evidence that moderate alcohol consumption helps preserve bone mass. A study done using sets of identical twins found that those who drank moderately had greater bone density at both the hip and spine than those who abstained. This may be partly due to alcohol's ability to boost estrogen levels.

Alcohol and Diabetes

According to Harvard Medical School, moderate wine consumption can reduce a woman's risk of developing type II diabetes. In the decade long study of premenopausal women, those who drank one or two glasses of red wine per day reduced their risk of developing the disease by approximately 40 percent.

Too Much of a Good Thing?

While there are some well documented health benefits derived from moderate alcohol consumption, drinking alcohol in large quantities can have devastating results. In 2006 it was determined that the life expectancy of Russian males was only 59 years and alcohol abuse was considered to be a contributing factor.

Alcohol and Vitamin Depletion

There is considerable evidence that excessive use of alcohol can seriously deplete your body's supply of certain vitamins and minerals, particularly vitamin C and potassium. In addition, large quantities of alcohol block calcium and thiamin absorption, as well as your body's ability to utilize vitamin D.

Alcohol and Obesity

While the term "beer belly" is a part of our culture, most people don't realize how many calories alcohol actually contains. Each gram has seven calories, almost double the four in a gram of protein or carbohydrates. Below are calorie counts for a number of popular beverages. This information might help you make a choice your waistline can live with.

Good Choices

Light Beer: This popular beverage has only 80-100 calories in a twelve ounce bottle. For many people a beer lasts longer than many sweet drinks that have considerably more calories. This helps cut down on total intake. Great commercials too!

Wine: In addition to the well documented health benefits that red wine provides, a four-ounce glass, the typical serving size, contains only about 90-100 calories. While white wine and champagne offer less health benefit, the calorie count is similar.

Cocktails with 80 proof vodka: One ounce of vodka contains about 65 calories. Since the average cocktail has about one-and-a-half ounces of liquor, vodka combined with water or club soda is a good choice when trying to keep one's figure. Fruit juice adds calories but with some nutritional value. The addition of sugary liquors tips the scale in the wrong direction (literally!).

Bad Choices

Liqueurs: These drinks are all sugar and have the calories to prove it. While the exact totals vary considerably, many contain over 100 calories per ounce, with Southern Comfort and Creme de Menthe weighing in at over 120. To add to the problem, the sweet flavor of these beverages often leads consumers to drink them more quickly than they would a less tasty drink. This frequently leads to greater total consumption.

Margaritas: This popular drink is a combination of tequila, triple sec and lime juice. Margaritas often include some sort of sugary flavoring, which can push its calorie total up to 400 or more. Adding salt around the rim can have a negative impact on blood pressure.

Pina Coladas: While a 7.5-ounce gin and tonic contains only 171 calories a 4.5-ounce pina colada weighs in at a hefty 262, that's just over half the drink for one and a half times the calories.

Daiquiris: For those who are counting calories daiquiris are also a poor choice. An eight ounce daiquiri contains approximately 430 calories, more than four times the total in four ounces of wine or twelve ounces of light beer.

Snacks: No, these aren't drinks, but they often accompany them on their way to your ever-expanding midsection. Hot dogs, pretzels and potato chips might make a football game seem complete, but unless you plan on playing a few downs at the end of the day to help burn them off, you will probably be letting your belt out a notch or two.

Alcohol and Brain Cells

It is considered a fact that alcohol kills brain cells. Brain cells do not regenerate so once you lose them—that's it! Studies have also found the brains, specifically the prefrontal cortices, of teenage drinkers to be smaller than those who do not drink.

Alcohol and Cancer

Studies have shown that alcohol significantly increases the risk of developing oral or breast cancer. Heather Spencer Feigelson, PhD., of the American Cancer Society states, "Alcohol consumption is associated with an increased risk of breast cancer." That view is echoed by Dr. Christine Horner, author of the book *Waking the Warrior Goddess*. Dr. Horner lists alcohol as a contributing factor in the two to three million cases of breast cancer currently afflicting the American population.

Alcohol and Blood Pressure

There is clear evidence that excessive alcohol intake is a primary contributor to high blood pressure. Alcohol can also decrease the effectiveness of some blood-pressure medications as well as increase their side effects.

Alcohol and Menopause

The typical age for the onset of menopause is between 48 and 55, however, menopausal symptoms sometimes begin up to ten years earlier. One of the factors in the early onset of menopause is a high level of alcohol consumption. This is due to alcohol's tendency to weaken the body, thereby causing it to cease some of its normal functions. A symptom of early menopause is difficulty controlling the bladder. This too is exacerbated by alcohol intake, due to its tendency to increase the frequency of urination.

An Exercise

Many people do not realize just how much they drink. Since overdoing it is clearly not a healthy choice, here's an exercise that can prove helpful. Make a chart of the next four weeks and keep it somewhere visible. Next, make a chart of the week ahead, small enough to carry in your wallet or purse. Examples of both charts are printed on the following pages so that you can copy them if you like. For the next four weeks, list exactly what alcoholic beverages you consume on the weekly calendars. At the end of each week transfer the info onto your monthly chart. For example, today's log entry might read: three glasses of wine and two beers or one beer and two mixed drinks. Put a red mark on any day where you have had more than the one to two drinks that medical science has shown to be beneficial. Review the chart weekly, then again at the end of the month. If you list your intake accurately you might be surprised at just how much alcohol you're putting into your body.

SAMPLE WEEK

	SUNDAY	MONDAY	TUESDAY	WEDNESDAY	THURSDAY	FRIDAY	SATURDAY
L	L //	L	L	L	L	L ///	L
B	B	B	B	B	B	B	B
W	W	W	W	W //	W /	W //	W
M	M	M	M	M	M	M //	M

ONE WEEK

	SUNDAY	MONDAY	TUESDAY	WEDNESDAY	THURSDAY	FRIDAY	SATURDAY
L	L	L	L	L	L	L	L
B	B	B	B	B	B	B	B
W	W	W	W	W	W	W	W
M	M	M	M	M	M	M	M

ONE WEEK

	SUNDAY	MONDAY	TUESDAY	WEDNESDAY	THURSDAY	FRIDAY	SATURDAY
L	L	L	L	L	L	L	L
B	B	B	B	B	B	B	B
W	W	W	W	W	W	W	W
M	M	M	M	M	M	M	M

L — Light Beer   B — Beer   W — Wine   M — Mixed Drink

FOUR WEEKS

WEEK 1

	SUNDAY	MONDAY	TUESDAY	WEDNESDAY	THURSDAY	FRIDAY	SATURDAY
L							
B							
W							
M							

WEEK 2

	SUNDAY	MONDAY	TUESDAY	WEDNESDAY	THURSDAY	FRIDAY	SATURDAY
L							
B							
W							
M							

WEEK 3

	SUNDAY	MONDAY	TUESDAY	WEDNESDAY	THURSDAY	FRIDAY	SATURDAY
L							
B							
W							
M							

WEEK 4

	SUNDAY	MONDAY	TUESDAY	WEDNESDAY	THURSDAY	FRIDAY	SATURDAY
L							
B							
W							
M							

Another Exercise

I know a woman who has a limited tolerance for alcohol but enjoys having a few now and then. She came up with a pretty good game plan to help keep her intake under control. When she heads out on the town for some socializing she wears a ring on each finger of her right hand. Every time she has a drink she moves one over to the left. Since she knows that three drinks is her limit, this keeps her from going overboard and ruining an otherwise fun night.

Want More Info?

For more information on the positive effects of moderate alcohol consumption visit Alcohol in Moderation's website at: www.aim-digest.com.

*"Thank God for tea! What would the world do without tea?
How did it exist? I am glad I was not born before tea."*
—English curate, Sidney Smith

30 9:30 p.m.
Will You Have A Cup Of Green Tea?

There is growing evidence that tea, in particular green tea, can help prevent a variety of health problems. According to John Weisburger, PhD, senior researcher at the Institute for Cancer Prevention in Valhalla, N.Y, tea modifies the metabolism to detoxify harmful chemicals. Based on these and other findings it seems safe to say that drinking a few cups of green tea each day is a good idea.

Health Benefits

*"If you are cold, tea will warm you; if you
are too heated, it will cool you;
if you are depressed, it will cheer you; if you
are excited, it will calm you."*
—William Ewart Gladstone

Tea and Cancer

In a study conducted at UCLA and reported in the February 15, 2005 issue of *Clinical Cancer Research*, green tea was found to target cancer cells without harming healthy tissue. According to Jian Yu Rao, MD, "In effect, the green tea extract may keep the cancer cells confined and localized, where they are easier to treat and the prognosis is better."

According to Dr. Christine Horner, author of, *Waking the Warrior Goddess*, green tea is a powerful weapon in the fight against breast cancer. Other studies have shown that green tea prevents the growth of certain tumors, thereby lowering the risk of prostate and other cancers. This is due in part to the high concentration of antioxidants called polyphenols that are found in tea.

Tea and Cholesterol

Numerous studies have noted the ability of green tea to lower cholesterol levels. In a Japanese study, more than 13,000 people drank one cup of green tea per day. The positive effect on cholesterol levels was considered significant. There is evidence that in addition to lowering total cholesterol, tea may raise levels of HDL.

Tea and Osteoporosis

Bone density is a major concern as we age, especially for women. Studies have shown that women who drink tea have greater bone density than those who do not. Benefits were most notable in those individuals who had been drinking tea for at least six years.

Tea and Heart Disease

In May 2006, an article was published in the *Journal of the American College of Surgeons* that lauded green tea's ability to combat heart disease. Lead author Bauer Sumpio, M.D., noted a correlation between a substance called epigallocatechin gallate, (EGCG), which is abundant in tea, and the low rate of heart disease in Asia.

Survival rates for those having already suffered a heart attack may also be improved by regular tea consumption. A study published in the American Heart Association's journal, *Circulation*, found that those who drink two or more cups of tea per day lowered their risk of death following a heart attack by 44 percent.

Tea and Your Teeth

Research has shown that drinking tea can protect your gums against the deterioration that often comes with aging. There is also evidence that the fluoride content in tea can help prevent tooth decay. On the downside, some teas can stain your teeth. Still, having white teeth doesn't help much if they are no longer in your mouth.

History

Who originated tea and how long it has been around is a matter of legend throughout the Orient. This popular beverage can be traced back to China nearly 5000 years ago. There, Shen Nung, a Chinese emperor, thought by many to be the father of Chinese herbal medicine, wrote about tea's thirst-quenching and energizing properties. Nung, sometimes referred to as "The Divine Healer", praised the ability of tea to treat a number of different ailments including tumors and conditions affecting the bladder.

Types of Tea

Whether black, white, oolong or green, all tea comes from the same plant, *Camellia sinensis*. What separates one type from another is the amount of processing. Green tea has less than its cousins, black and oolong, and as a result has greater health benefits. While white has less still, its high price and lesser availability, makes green the tea of choice for those seeking its beneficial effects rather than just its flavor.

Herbal Teas (Tisanes)

Technically speaking, these popular beverages are not actually tea. Herbal teas, also known as tisanes, are not the product of the *Camellia sinensis*, but instead are brewed from the parts of an assortment of plants which are capable of producing a tea-like beverage. Since they are not made from the same plant, it follows that the health benefits that herbal teas provide may be markedly different or even non-existent. Still, people crave products with buzzwords like "natural", "organic" and "herbal." As a result, herbal teas continue to enjoy a great deal of popularity and a place on the shelves of supermarkets and health food stores nationwide.

What's in the Bag?

When looking at a tea bag it is difficult to visualize the healing power contained within. Below is a brief analysis of several healthful compounds that are found in green tea. Reading about them will help you to understand the benefits that this beverage provides.

Flavonoids

These naturally occurring substances are believed to possess antioxidant properties. They are present in tea and help fight cancer and some viruses. They are also believed to be both antiallergic and anti-inflammatory.

Quercetin: A flavonoid that is plentiful in tea. Quercetin has demonstrated both anti-inflammatory and antioxidant properties, making it effective in combating a wide variety of ailments including arthritis, fibromyalgia, cancer, cataracts and macular degeneration. Since quercetin also acts as an antihistamine, allergy sufferers may benefit from increasing their consumption of this compound.

Catechin: A flavonoid that is a natural antibiotic and is abundant in both black and green tea. Catechin has been shown to lower the risk of heart disease. There is also evidence that this compound may inhibit tumor growth, making it a potent cancer-fighting agent. Catechin is also beneficial to those suffering from diarrhea.

Polyphenols

These compounds found in tea leaves, have been shown to possess antioxidant properties. According to the National Cancer Institute, they also, "...may reduce abnormal cell growth and inflammation; help the body get rid of cancer-causing agents; and restore communication between different cells in the body." There is some evidence that polyphenols may block the intestinal absorption of cholesterol, thereby lowering your risk of heart disease.

Tannins: Present in tea, coffee, red wine, walnuts and pomegranates, tannins have been shown to be beneficial when taken in concentrations that are moderate. In high concentrations, however, they can inhibit the body's ability to absorb iron and other minerals.

Theanine

Theanine is an amino acid that is found in tea. It produces a feeling of relaxation by increasing the brain's levels of serotonin and dopamine. Some studies have shown theanine to be an immune booster.

How Long Should You Brew?

Tea that you steep is considered to be far more beneficial than the varieties sold in bottles or cans. To gain the full health benefits it is generally recommended to let your tea steep for a full three to five minutes prior to drinking.

How Much Should You Drink?

Keep in mind that while only one cup of tea is written into your daily planner, multiple cups are recommended. Having a cup with each meal is a good way to increase your intake. This increased consumption will enable you to enjoy tea's full benefits.

Don't Believe the Hype

The data supporting the value of green tea seems valid. Still, the outrageous promises made by unscrupulous tea peddlers cast doubt on what is clearly a quality product. Statements like: "Lose ten pounds in six weeks, I will guarantee it!" detract from what green tea can really do for you when consumed on a regular basis. Always be wary of outrageous claims regarding tea or any other product.

Tea Tips

*Hold the Milk: There is some evidence that caseins, proteins found in milk, may reduce the cardiovascular health benefits that tea provides.

*Add a Wedge of Lemon: The juice of this popular fruit helps cleanse the body of toxins. In addition, the high vitamin C content of lemon helps to reverse one of the few negative aspects of tea consumption, its tendency to block the absorption of iron consumed from non-animal sources.

*Hold the Sugar: The harmful effects of sugar have been well documented. Too much added sugar can offset many of the benefits that tea provides.

*Add a Cinnamon Stick: As we read in chapter seven, this flavorful herb may help to regulate both blood sugar and cholesterol levels.

Interesting Fact

Tea is the second most popular drink in the world, surpassed only by water. In the United States, however, it comes in sixth trailing not only water but also coffee, soda, beer and milk.

Suggested Reading

The Book of Green Tea by Diana Rosen (Storey Publishing, LLC January, 1998)

Green Tea by Nadine Taylor (Kensington Publishing Corporation (January 1998)

Want More Info?

For those seeking further information on what tea has to offer the Tea Association of the United States of America has an excellent website. Visit them at: www.teausa.com.

In addition, author and tea expert Diana Rosen publishes a monthly newsletter that contains a wealth of information on the topic. Visit her website at: www.teamuse.com.

"It is impossible to list all the kinds of good sex. There are too many."
—The Kama Sutra

31 | 11 p.m.
Will You Have Sex?

In January 2005, *The Bedroom Workout for Men*, a DVD that I created, went on sale. It's an exercise program that will get you in shape for sex. The question remains, is sex in itself good exercise? The answer, happily, is yes. Sex, assuming it is safe, is as healthy an activity as it is an enjoyable one. It relieves stress, burns calories and gives many muscle groups a thorough workout.

Health Benefits

"Sex, that's life, man."
—Fitness Guru Jack LaLanne at 91

Sex and Cardiovascular Fitness

In his classic, *Eat To Win*, Dr. Robert Haas' points out the cardiovascular value of a spirited romantic encounter. Dr. Haas compares the physiological changes brought about by vigorous sex—rapid heart rate, elevated blood pressure and profuse sweating—with playing tennis or running a marathon. A British study also pointed out that regular sex can lead to a healthy heart. The study followed 900 men and found that those who had sex at least twice each week reduced their risk of having a heart attack.

Sex and Calorie Expenditure

The next question in our weight conscious society is obvious, how many calories does sex actually burn? To accurately calculate calorie expenditure, you must first determine the person's heart rate. Research shows that a healthy individual who is taking the less active role during sexual activity often remains between 120 and 130 beats per minute. The same is true of those who are in a non-weight-bearing position (lying down). When assuming a more active role, or when in a weight-bearing position, an individual's heart rate often reaches or exceeds the mid-140s. This is due to the energy requirements of increased movement as well as the effects of gravity.

Assuming the person we're talking about is working at the higher level (mid-140s), that would be equivalent to somewhere between a typical aerobics class and running at a moderate pace (aerobics burns approximately 5 calories per kilogram of bodyweight per hour, while running burns about 7). Assuming an average of 6 and a woman of 120 pounds, which equals 54.545 kilograms, she would burn about 327.27 calories per hour of sex. At the slower pace, we might liken the intensity to rapid walking (a pace of about 4 MPH). Here many women reach a heart rate in the mid-120s and burn about 3.4 cal. per kg per hour, (about 185.453 calories per hour).

For a 200 pound man, (90.72kg) we would use the same formula, 544.32 calories per hour at the faster pace as compared with 308.5 calories per hour at the lower level of intensity. During the sprint towards the goal line many people may achieve, or even exceed, the 160 BPM mentioned by Dr. Haas.

For those who are young, healthy, and maintain a reasonable bodyweight, this is usually a performance concern not one of health. However, for individuals who are older, obese, or who have cardiorespiratory issues, sex can be dangerous and occasionally fatal—so stay in shape!

Sex and Stress Reduction

One of the greatest benefits that regular sex provides is its ability to relieve stress. While stress reduction has a strong emotional component, physiological factors should not be overlooked. One such factor is the increased level of a hormone called oxytocin that occurs during orgasm. Oxytocin, a hormone secreted by the pituitary gland, plays a role in stress reduction as well as many other physiological functions.

Sex and Fertility

In the 1970s studies were done by Dr. Winifred Cutler, the results of which were interesting to many in the medical community. They showed that women who had heterosexual sex on a regular basis were more fertile. The evidence pointed to sex causing a delay in the decline of their level of estrogen.

Sex and an Enlarged Prostate

Benign prostatic hyperplasia or BPH is the technical term for a condition that many men are all too familiar with. It refers to an enlargement of the prostate that afflicts four out of five men by the age of seventy. While some prostate enlargement is inevitable, the severity of symptoms can vary. One thing that seems to help is regular sexual activity. In his book, *Live Now, Age Later*, Isadore Rosenfeld, M.D. states that, "Regular ejaculations ease congestion of the prostate."

Sex and Prostate Cancer

A Harvard University study found a link between frequent sexual activity and a lower risk of prostate cancer. It claimed that men who ejaculate 20 times or more per month have a prostate cancer rate 33 percent lower than those who do not. Another study conducted at Bethesda Maryland's National Cancer Center followed a group of 30,000 American men and produced similar results. Though the reason for this link has not been established, there are several theories as to why it may exist, including stress reduction and a cleansing of built up toxins.

Sex and Endometriosis

Endometriosis is a condition that affects over five million American women. This condition whose symptoms include pelvic and lower back pain, can lead to infertility. For those suffering from endometriosis the lesions that are symptomatic of this ailment can result in pain during intercourse, a symptom known as dyspareunia. Paradoxically, studies have shown that having sex on a regular basis may be an effective means of prevention.

Sex and Arthritis

Arthritis pain can make performing sexually more of a challenge. Still, for those who stick it out there is often an unexpected benefit, a reduction in arthritis pain. This is due in part to the increase in endorphin levels that sex produces. Endorphins, chemical compounds produced by the hypothalamus and pituitary glands, are natural pain killers.

Better Safe than Sorry

In a book that is dedicated to health and longevity I would be remiss not to mention the importance of keeping your sexual experience safe and disease free. When I was growing up condoms were the exception rather than the rule. The 70s and 80s were wild times and most sexually active women had discovered their birth control method of choice. Then the permanence of herpes got people's attention followed by the AIDS epidemic. In 2005, 3.1 million people died of AIDS worldwide with another 40.3 million infected. All of a sudden, rubber was back in vogue. Everyone makes their own choices in life but my suggestion here is to be smart. It's much easier to enjoy something once you take the risk out of the equation, especially when the consequences are this dire.

How Long do Condoms Last?

Most of us agree that condoms are necessary, but unlike true love, they won't last forever. Most reputable brands supply you with an expiration date. Remember to check it. While most condoms are good for up to five years, don't press your luck with the ones you left in the drawer back in high school.

Sex-Enhancing Supplements

In no segment of the highly lucrative supplement market are consumers as shamelessly preyed upon as they are in the area of enhanced sexual performance. From the dawn of time people have gobbled up everything from rhinoceros horn to truffles in a sometimes desperate attempt to improve their sexual performance. Yet, while much of what is promised is purely fiction, some supplements can be helpful, depending on the individual's specific circumstance. Below are several that you might consider, along with some info that can help you choose to either use them or pass them by.

Zinc: We've all heard the legend of oysters and improved sexual performance. As with most old wives tales it contains a grain of truth. Back when most people's diets were far more limited than they are today, many men suffered from sterility and/or impotence due to a lack of zinc. Oysters are rich in zinc. The great minds of the time found that by eating oysters those rather undesirable problems would go away. Today most people's diets are more diverse. Still, zinc deficiencies are not as rare as you might suspect and those symptoms still exist to one degree or another. Therefore, if good sexual performance is your goal, than making sure that your diet contains adequate levels of zinc is still a pretty good idea.

Zinc supplements are another matter, and the potential for toxicity should not be ignored. Doses ranging from 100-300 mg per day have been shown to impair immune function as well as the body's ability to utilize copper. Quality multivitamins usually contain 15 mg of zinc, 100 percent of the RDA. This total should be adequate for most people's needs. For those who choose to supplement, make sure to take no more than 100 mg per day, unless directed by a physician. Also be aware that those suffering from sexual dysfunction not related to a zinc deficiency are unlikely to gain relief from zinc supplementation.

Ginseng: Everyone is familiar with the sex enhancing reputation of this oddly shaped root. But can we believe the hype? The answer here, as with zinc, depends on what is causing the problem. Ginseng is considered an ergogenic aid, a substance that boosts your energy level. If your lack of prowess is due to low energy then ginseng might prove helpful. However, if your poor performance has a different cause then it's unlikely that ginseng will help. Also bear in mind that ginseng, like all supplements, is not currently regulated by the FDA. When ConsumerLab.com performed a study of 22 popular brands it found that eight of them contained unhealthy levels of pesticides while others were contaminated with lead.

Yohimbine: Made from the bark of a tree native to Africa, yohimbine has been touted as an effective treatment for erectile dysfunction. In studies performed at both Kingston General Hospital and Ontario's Queen's University, improvement was seen in over 40 percent of those tested.

Yohimbine is sold both as an over-the-counter herbal supplement and by doctor's prescription. Keep in mind that yohimbine has been known to raise blood pressure, so those with or prone to hypertension should probably not take this supplement. Other potential side effects include anxiety and insomnia.

Remember to always check with your physician before taking any supplement to make sure it won't either impact an existing condition or interfere with a medication being used to control one. Also keep in mind that with any drug or supplement the placebo effect cannot be discounted in regard to benefits received. However, if the potion is ruled safe and the results are good, do you really care why it worked?

In closing this chapter, it is worthwhile to point out that a spirited sexual encounter helps many people sleep, thereby preparing us for our final component.

Suggested Reading

The Practical Encyclopedia of Sex and Health by Steven Bechtel (Rodale Books, April 1993)

"There is a time for many words, and there is also a time for sleep."
—Homer

"Oh sleep! It is a gentle thing, Beloved from pole to pole."
—Samuel Taylor Coleridge

32 Midnight How Much Sleep Will You Get?

A long day has come to an end and it's time to get some sleep. Studies have shown that people who sleep too little live shorter lives. Surprisingly, the same reports show similar results for those who sleep too much. In general it's safe to say that seven to eight hours a night is optimal. This allows your body time to adequately repair itself.

As with exercise, there is more to consider than just duration. Quality of sleep is as important as quantity and is affected by many factors. Sleep can be enhanced by creating a relaxing bedtime environment through the use of a pleasing fragrance, soothing music and a comfortable room temperature. Having the right sheets and pillows also work to facilitate a good night's sleep, as does having a comfortable mattress. Factors that can negatively affect sleep patterns include stress as well as eating or consuming alcohol, caffeine or nicotine within an hour or two before bed.

Your Mattress

Here is a brain teaser for you: Name something you spend one third of your life on but pay almost no attention to? Give up? It's your mattress. While your mattress is a big part of how well you sleep, unless their back is aching most people don't think much about it. There are two questions you should ask yourself: what model should I buy and at what point should I replace it?

Choosing a Mattress

Since its development in eighteenth century Europe, the innerspring mattress has made sleep a great deal more comfortable. Still, choosing one can be a stressful and confusing experience. According to *Consumer Reports*, they receive more inquiries about mattresses than any product other than cars:

> "The reason is that shoppers are flying blind. It's hard to tell one box of metal, foam, fuzz, and fabric from another, making you vulnerable to a sales pitch. Model names differ from store to store, making it impossible to comparison shop, and prices vary so much that the $1,300 mattress set you look at one day can cost $2,600 the next."

One Lump or Two: When to Change Your Mattress

Your mattress should not overstay its welcome. Not only will it lose support, but over time a mattress can double in weight, due to an accumulation of body oils, dead skin, dust mites and perspiration. A general rule of thumb is to replace mattresses that have no box spring about once every ten years, or when you see evidence of sagging. As for mattresses with a box spring, the lifespan can be extended another two or three years.

Buying Tip

Purchases are often made on impulse or as the result of an aggressive salesperson. To avoid making a mistake that will keep you up nights, make sure that your new mattress has a 30-day money-back guarantee.

Sheets

Choose sheets made from 100% cotton. While products containing polyester or acrylic plastics are available, your body heat may cause them to emit toxic gasses that can irritate both your skin and eyes. Also steer clear of sheets labeled "easy-care" or "permanent press". Such products may be treated with formaldehyde, a known carcinogen.

While you can keep your sheets for quite a while you should change and launder them every week, two weeks at the most. The reason is little creatures called dust mites that live in your bedding, feeding on dead skin cells. The only proven way to kill them is to launder your sheets in hot water, ideally over 130 degrees.

Pillows

The first decision when selecting pillows is whether they will be filled with feathers or man made materials. The choice is not always a matter of taste. For those with asthma or weakened immune systems, feathered pillows are often a far better option than those made of synthetic substances. This is because of the many species of fungus that flourish in the environment that synthetic fibers provide. These tiny organisms that are not harmful to many of us can be a health hazard to that segment of the population and should therefore be avoided.

The approximate lifespan of your pillows is between one and three years. At that point the pressure placed on them each night may have resulted in reduced head and neck support. Examine your pillows periodically for lumps and if you find them, do some shopping.

All the Bells and Whistles

When I was in my early 20s, a high pressure salesman talked my normally frugal mother into buying a bed just slightly less expensive than the family car. It had all the features one could ask for; you could raise your head or feet, heat it or make it vibrate, all with the touch of a button. It was something new and she enjoyed it at first but didn't seem to sleep any better. Soon the novelty wore off. Then some features stopped working altogether. Over the years it began to deteriorate as any bed would but the high price caused her to hang onto it long after it should have been retired. This is not meant as an indictment of such products. Still, you should always be aware of the pitfalls before purchasing an item whose cost keeps you awake long after its vibrating fingers should have worked their magic.

Melatonin

A hormone produced in the pineal gland, melatonin is a key player in our sleep cycle. Its secretion is stimulated by dark and inhibited by light. Since levels of melatonin tend to decrease with age, sleep can become more elusive. If this is the case, then melatonin supplements can help. They are available in both pill and lozenge form and doses between .5 mg and 12mg are recommended for those wishing to regulate their sleep cycle. As with any supplement there are potential side effects so it is best to consult your physician before beginning a program of melatonin supplementation.

Sleeping Pills

When sleep remains elusive some people resort to sleeping pills. While effective, these drugs, whether bought over the counter or obtained by prescription, often cause more problems than they solve. This is especially true for the elderly. The side effects include worsening the symptoms of asthma, glaucoma or an enlarged prostate. These medications also cause dry mouth and are often habit forming. Think twice before relying on this "quick fix." Taken regularly it might give you something to really lose sleep over.

Sleep and Obesity

A study done in 2004 at New York's Columbia University opened quite a few eyes to the value of shutting them. It found that those who slept four to six hours a night faced a much higher risk of obesity than those better rested. Individuals who slept less than six hours a night increased their risk by 23 percent, while those who sleep less than four hours a night face a 73 percent greater risk of obesity. It was also found that people who sleep ten or more hours a day are 11 percent less likely to be obese.

A great deal of research on this topic revolves around a hormone called leptin. Produced by the body's fat cells, leptin's functions include initiating the burning of calories and suppressing the appetite. Sleep deprivation has been shown to decrease leptin levels, thereby *increasing* appetite.

Another hormone receiving a great deal of attention is ghrelin. Lack of sleep causes ghrelin levels to rise, causing feelings of hunger. A correlation has been found between high levels of ghrelin and obesity.

Sleep Disorders

"Sleeplessness is a desert without vegetation or inhabitants."
—Jessamyn West

Sleep disorders affect the lives of 40 million Americans. Below are some conditions that can affect the length and quality of sleep as well as a number of symptoms that may result from those conditions. Treatment options are also listed. By educating yourself to the potential problems that exist, you can identify and seek treatment for those that apply to you. By doing so, sleep and the benefits that come from it can be enhanced.

Sleep Apnea

Complicating the sleep/obesity connection is a condition known as sleep apnea, an ailment that affects over twelve million Americans. While as we have seen too little sleep can lead to obesity, obesity itself can result in this serious and potentially life threatening condition that causes those affected to stop breathing as they sleep. Sleep apnea can lead to a variety of ailments including high blood pressure and heart disease and is considered the cause of many motor vehicle accidents. For some sufferers, weight loss alone can solve the problem. For others, a blockage in the airway is the cause. Treatment options often include the use of a mask system known as C-Pap.

Narcolepsy

A neurological disorder that affects more than one in every 2000 Americans, narcolepsy can easily turn the sufferer's life upside down. According to Dr. Alcibiades Rodriguez of the New York Sleep Institute, "The essential feature of narcolepsy is the intrusion of REM sleep during wakefulness (paralysis) and wakefulness in REM sleep (hallucinations upon falling asleep and waking up)." Narcolepsy can be diagnosed through the use of a Polysomnogram (PSG) and a Multiple Sleep Latency Test (MSLT). Treatment options include stimulants to relieve excessive daytime sleepiness. Medications that stimulate norepinephrine release are also given for the treatment of cataplexy, a symptom of narcolepsy. Be aware that the effectiveness of these drugs varies from one person to another, as do the side effects. According to Dr. Rodriguez, "The treatment aims to correct the symptoms and scientists are still working on the primary causes of narcolepsy."

Cataplexy

A phenomenon characterized by a sudden loss of muscle tone. For those suffering from narcolepsy, this symptom is often brought on by emotions such as laughter, fear or anger. While they do not lose consciousness, those suffering a cataleptic attack will often lie motionless for several minutes until normal functioning returns.

Sleep Paralysis

Often a symptom of narcolepsy, this phenomenon occurs in up to 40 percent of young adults. Sleep paralysis is characterized by the temporary inability to move or speak while falling asleep (predormital) or while waking up (postdormital).

Insomnia

Sometimes the sleep that you crave eludes you. This can be the result of many factors including anxiety, the use of stimulants and some health problems. After a while, you start to worry about not getting to sleep, which makes doing so even more difficult. There are as many solutions to this problem as there are causes. Some useful suggestions are listed under "sleep tips" at the end of this chapter.

Restless Leg Syndrome

Restless leg syndrome (RLS) is a neurological disorder that afflicts approximately ten percent of the American population. RLS is characterized by an irresistible urge to move your legs that starts or grows worse when resting. The discomfort is greatest in the evening and is often accompanied by uncomfortable sensations. Temporary relief can be attained by moving the affected limb.

Drugs are an option in treating RLS but other approaches have also proven affective. They include, eating a balanced diet, vitamin supplementation, exercise and eliminating caffeine and/or alcohol consumption. Those affected should consult their physician to find the treatment plan that is best for them. The Restless Leg Foundation also has a helpful website. It is located at: www.rls.org.

Other Factors

Nightmares

Nightmares are disturbing dreams that result in emotional distress. While individual nightmares are not dangerous, approximately ten percent of American adults suffer from trauma-inducing dreams on a regular basis. The causes of nightmares vary from person to person but include stress, traumatic life experiences and certain medications.

Treatment options include psychotherapy and various relaxation techniques. It is important to gain an understanding of the cause. By understanding the source of the problem, therapists can better select a treatment program.

Snoring

Most of us have been around a snorer at one time or another and have found it either annoying or amusing. Few, however, have thought of snoring as a health problem. According to Dr. Michael Gelb, a specialist in the field, "Every time you snore your brain wakes up." He estimates that 90 million Americans suffer from this affliction that can interfere with the quality of sleep. Snoring is caused by an interruption in the flow of air to the lungs, often the result of a nasal deformity that forms an obstruction. The obstruction causes a vibration of the surrounding tissue, resulting in the sounds with which we are familiar.

Numerous treatment options are available to those afflicted, depending on the cause of the problem. If obesity is a contributing factor then weight loss can help. If nasal congestion is the cause then nasal strips or various medications can help. Consult your physician to determine the treatment that is best for you.

The Role of Allergens

Allergies to a wide variety of substances affect over 40 million

Americans. Loss of sleep is a common result of many allergies. Ironically, allergies can rob you of the very sleep needed to reduce their symptoms. The effects of many of them can be combated by opening a window periodically and airing out your home. Home air filters can also help. The better ones can remove a wide assortment of irritants including mold, smoke and pet dander.

Recommendation

In order to lead a healthy, productive life, seven to eight hours of sleep a night, augmented by meditation, is ideal. For more on the benefits of meditation, refer back to chapters 1 and 19. When you sleep less, a nap can help make up for what you are missing. Make sure your mattress is comfortable and has not exceeded its lifespan. Finally, if you have any of the conditions described earlier in this chapter it may be advisable to consult a physician. Left untreated, small problems tend to become larger over time.

Better Sleep Tips

*Sound Machines: Sound in the form of "white noise" can often help when sleep has otherwise eluded you. Many models offer the ability to switch between a number of different soothing, repetitive sounds including wind, rain and waterfalls that can go on all night if you so desire. Some of the better models offer several options including rate, range and tone so that you can mix and match.

*Music: Recordings, while finite in length, can also be very effective. They offer a much greater variety of sounds, so that each individual can choose what works best for them. While some are soothed by actual music, others prefer whale sounds or waves crashing on the beach.

*Keep a Pad Handy: It is common at bedtime for our minds to race, thinking about all the things we'll need to do once we awake. Keeping a pad handy and writing thoughts down as they come to you will free your mind and allow you to relax.

*Keep the Room Comfy: This means different things to different people. Some enjoy sleeping in a toasty warm room, others prefer it cool. Whichever your preference, go the extra mile to get the temperature where you want it. Whether it's dragging an extra blanket out of the closet or prying open that sticky window, doing so will pay dividends once you settle under the covers.

*Don't Get Stressed: This sounds easier than it is, however, getting upset right before bed can kill the mood and keep you awake for hours.

Avoid dwelling on matters that trouble you. Instead, fill the end of your day with soothing music, gentle fragrances and tranquil thoughts.

*Visualization: Picturing yourself in a situation that you find soothing is a great way to help you drift off. Some obvious choices are lounging on a sandy beach while listening to the waves roll in or relaxing in a grassy meadow with a cool breeze blowing gently by.

*Stick to a Schedule: Inconsistent bedtime schedules are a contributing factor to a number of sleep disorders, especially for the elderly. An example of this is the phenomenon called "jet lag" where a sudden change in time zones forces sleep patterns to adjust, leaving the individual feeling lethargic and irritable. Going to bed at the same time every night can help those who find sleep hard to come by.

*Use a Night-Light: Bright light can reduce your level of melatonin. Exposure for even a few minutes can make falling back asleep more difficult. If you're someone who wakes up in the middle of the night for a drink of water or a trip to the bathroom, consider having night-lights in the appropriate rooms. Doing so will enable you to return to sleep as quickly as possible.

*Hold a Piece of Amethyst: Amethyst is a type of quartz that is often purple in color. Many within the holistic health community believe that amethyst can be helpful to those suffering from insomnia. If sleep proves elusive, try holding February's birthstone in your hand, or place one inside your pillowcase.

Suggested Reading

The Promise of Sleep by William C. Dement and Christopher Vaughan (Dell, March 7, 2000)

Sleep Disorders for Dummies by Max Hirshkowitz, PhD and Patricia B. Smith (For Dummies, May 7, 2004)

Want More Info?

For more information on the subject of sleep, the National Sleep Foundation has an excellent website. Visit them at: www.sleepfoundation.org.

For more information on sleep disorders visit the website of the National Center on Sleep Disorders Research at: www.nhlbi.nih.gov/about/ncsdr.

"If you think you can do a thing or think you can't do a thing, you're right."
—Henry Ford

A Closing Word or Two

The above day is just a guideline, as people's schedules vary widely. Some work across the street from the gym and two blocks from home, while others have a two hour commute. Still, these concepts are valid and if followed, might improve the length and quality of your life. Try incorporating them into your daily routine.

Also keep in mind that a positive attitude is viewed by many anti-aging experts as the single most important factor in maintaining your youth and vitality. I did not include a separate section on that topic, since it should always be with you as an integral part of your personality.

Finally, join me in paying tribute to the people of Andorra, the tiny nation bordering Spain whose citizens currently enjoy the world's longest life expectancy, 83.5 years.

Bibliography

Below is a list of books on this topic too general to have been included at the end of the previous chapters. They contain a wealth of useful information and many of them have been helpful in accumulating the knowledge necessary to create this book; many thanks to their authors for helping us to live longer and better.

American Council on Exercise. *Personal Trainer Manual.* San Diego, CA: American Council on Exercise, 1996

Bruun, Ruth Dowling, M.D., and Bruun, Bertel, M.D. *THE Human Body.* New York: Random House, 1982

Buhner, Stephen Harrod. *Herbal Antibiotics. Pownal,* VT: Storey Books, 1999

Carper, Jean. *Stop Aging Now!.* New York: HarperCollins, 1996

Edstrom, Krs. *Healthy Wealthy & Wise.* Los Angeles, CA: Soft Stone Publishing, 1999

Kapit, Wynn and Elson, Lawrence M. *The Anatomy Coloring Book.* New York: HarperCollins, 1997

Klatz, Ronald Dr., and Goldman, Robert Dr. *Stopping The Clock.* North Bergen, NJ: Basic Health Publications, Inc., 2002

Niven, David, Ph.D. *The 100 Simple Secrets of Healthy People.* New York: HarperCollins, 2003

Null, Gary, Ph.D. Gary Null's *Power Aging.* New York: New American Library, 2004

Pentz, Jane, Dr., *If You Don't Take Care Of Your Body Where Are You Going To Live.* West Roxbury, MA: LMA Publishing, 2004

Rosenfeld, Isadore, M.D. *Live Now, Age Later.* New York: Warner Books, 2000

Stoff, Jesse A., M.D., and Clouatre, Dallas, Ph.D. *The Prostate Miracle.* New York: Kensington Books, 2000

Index

R

S

WEEKLY CHART

Below is the weekly chart mentioned in the introduction. By copying it and placing it somewhere visible like on your refrigerator you can take a minute at the end of each day and check off the areas where you feel you've made the grade. On non exercise days put a circle through the three boxes that make up the fitness component.

	S	M	T	W	T	F	S
Did You Meditate?							
How Much Water Did You drink?							
Did You Try Aromatherapy?							
Have You Revised Your Wardrobe Lately?							
Did You Check Your Posture?							
How Often Did You Wash Your Hands?							
Did You Eat Breakfast?							
Did You Take a Multivitamin?							
Did You Use Sunscreen?							
Did You Start Your Day with Music?							
Did You Pet the Dog?							
Were You Stifled by Clutter?							
Did You Take the Stairs?							
How Did You Breathe?							
Did You Spend This Time Worrying?							
Did You Learn Something New?							
Were You Wishing Your Life Away?							
Did You Have a Midmorning Snack?							
When Was Your Last Massage?							
What Did You Have for Lunch?							
Did You Meditate Again?							
Did You Laugh?							
How Many Hours Did You Work?							
Did You Stretch?							
Did You Do Any Strength Training?							
Did You Do Cardio?							
What Was Your Second Snack?							
What Did You Have for Dinner?							
Did You Drink Alcohol and If So, How Much?							
Did You Have a Cup Of Green Tea?							
Did You Have Sex?							
How Much Sleep Did You Get?							